REBEL VEGAN LIFE

A PLANT-BASED NUTRITION AND BEGINNER'S GUIDE

TODD SINCLAIR

First published 2021 by Intrepid Fox Publishing Ltd

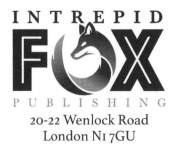

20-22 Wenlock Road
London N1 7GU

Hardback ISBN 978-1-7398490-5-4
Paperback ISBN 978-1-7398490-4-7
eISBN 978-1-7398490-3-0

REBELVEGANLIFE.COM

Original Illustrations by Cathy Brear
Recipe Development by Lara Schirkhorschidi

Other Images by Shutterstock

This book is dedicated to my parents, Alan & Elva,
who gave me the confidence and support to go out
into the world and find my way home again.

Exclusive Thank You Gift
for Rebel Vegan Readers:

FREE Download of Complimentary ebook

TOP 10 VEGAN SUPERFOODS
With Nutritional Guidelines and Recipes

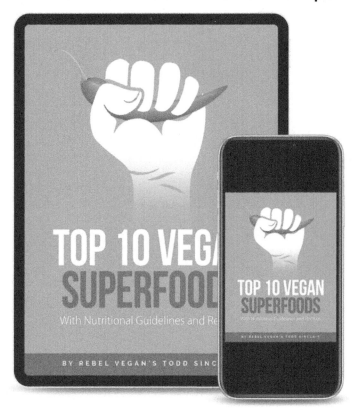

https://rebelveganlife.ck.page/rebelvegansuperfoods

CONTENTS

FOREWORD

The words "vegan" and "veganism" entered the lexicon in 1944. With that much history, you'd think that a plant-exclusive diet and cruelty-free lifestyle would be old hat – avant-garde, perhaps, when Great-Grandmother did it, but now, simply the way of the world. And yet, we're not there. We still need our rebels, and Todd Sinclair is stepping up as the James Dean of his generation, except that this rebel does indeed have a cause.

Rebel Vegan is a delightful and compelling read. It doesn't make its points by causing pre-vegans (or even ex-vegans) to feel bad about themselves, and yet it never falters from its conviction that this way of living is:

- Logical and accessible to most humans (certainly to you, as you read this book)
- Physiologically and nutritionally sound
- Environmentally crucial
- Ethically unassailable
- And in keeping with the teachings of the world's great wisdom traditions, even though you might not find vegan pastries at fellowship hour after church.

As Sinclair wrote this book, the timing meant that he was looking out on a world in turmoil. Climate Change is going forward, largely unabated. Politicians and their constituents are at such odds with one another, I wouldn't be surprised to see a controversy arise over the existence of gravity or the color of the sky. Many young people live for likes and wonder why life doesn't seem to mean much, while the majority of older people take multiple medications and have never been offered a lifestyle alternative to extend their "healthspan" and enjoy every decade.

In addition, we may well have entered the "Age of Epidemics," as our use and misuse of non-human animals makes us ready prey for zoonotic infections.

We could look at these, and the myriad other challenges we face, one at a time—creating more think tanks and forming more committees, raising more funds, and presenting more lectures—or we can take the rebel's stand: "I'm not waiting around for governments and corporations. I'm going to do something that will actually help, and I'm going to let everyone, in three dimensions or cyberspace, know what I'm doing and why." And what the rebels are doing is snubbing the status quo, thriving on a vegan lifestyle, and making some noise about it.

This is a courageous stand to take because it makes everything better: for animals, both human and other-than-human, for the planet, and for the future.

In these pages, Todd Sinclair invites all of us to become Rebel Vegans. Change overnight if that's your style, or start today and get this done in six months, or a year. Just don't turn back.

It's like stepping onto one of those moving walkways at an airport: you're going in the right direction, and before long, you'll be flying.

Victoria Moran

Author, Main Street Vegan
Host, Main Street Vegan Podcast

New York City, November 2021

victoria@mainstreetvegan.net

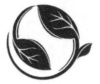

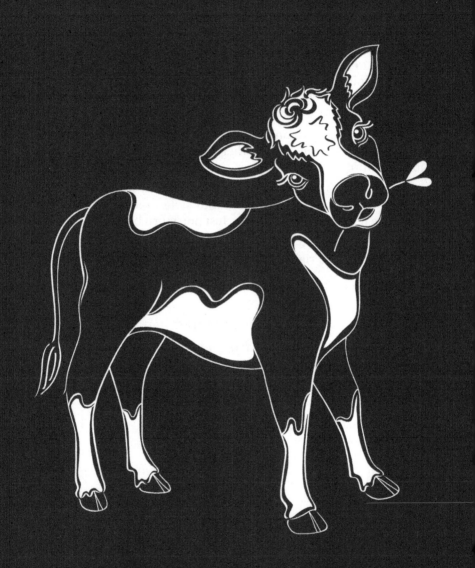

INTRODUCTION

REBEL'S HOMECOMING

"In a time of universal deceit - telling the truth is a revolutionary act."
GEORGE ORWELL[1]

Welcome home, fellow rebels.

Although veganism has become a buzzword and is breaking through into the mainstream consciousness, we are still the outsiders fighting for truth and compassion in a cruel and powerful system. Simply by being here, on page one, you are part of the solution and welcomed into our movement to create a kinder, refined future.

This book is all about celebrating, demystifying, and uncomplicating veganism to inspire and empower the rebel in us all. Inside are the keys to help you find your way with a complete plant-based nutritional guide and a flexible 4-step program to reduce or exclude animal products in an easy and lasting way. I also share all my secrets and stories for a successful sustainable life. We are all rebels here.

However, this is not a typical how-to guide, because you are not just another vegan. We all have our own unique relationship with food and must forge our own path to a more sustainable and healthy life. I see it as a homecoming to our original, authentic, caring selves. We all must find the compassion and truth inside us, and this book is a safe space to explore these different paths and find your way home. To be aligned with your values and build your best life.

Your journey towards a more sustainable, healthier lifestyle does not have to be difficult, nor should it include guilt trips or restrictions. I am not the vegan police. I promise never to preach, shame, or condescend. I will walk with you through this journey, offering inspiration and practical tips every step of the way.

The *REBEL VEGAN LIFE* ethos is about expanding your horizons and revealing new possibilities, not restricting them. Many people feel put off from adopting a vegan lifestyle because of the judgment or in-fighting that is, unfortunately, part of any movement. I appreciate that this may lead to many people turning away or feeling alienated from learning more, making better choices, and being more involved. I aim to open up the vegan space and welcome everyone to my table.

We cannot ignore that our diet and our health are linked. Eating meat and dairy leads to a greater likelihood of obesity, coronary heart disease, high blood pressure, cancer, and the development of zoonotic diseases.[2] And it's important to remember that humans are not carnivores by nature, but rather omnivores. We evolved, survived, and thrived on a primarily plant-based diet. Our diet is a choice. Our taste buds are habitual. It is an empowering and profound realization that changing our diets can bring so many benefits to ourselves and the world around us.

I am both a rebel and a realist. So, I am proposing a new way to go vegan. To make lasting change, we need to stay connected - to each other and to our shared values of compassion and justice. If we can support each other and embrace a life in line with these essential ethics, we can find our way home and solve many issues facing our world today.

So, *REBEL VEGAN* is a safe space for everyone—one where even mindful meat-eaters are welcome to pull a seat up to the table and learn what all the fuss is about. Anyone open to exploring the vegan world can find something that resonates or motivates them to make positive changes. So let's join the compassionate revolution.

If you are going to rebel, do it with purpose.

*"The inside of my fridge used to look like a morgue.
Now it is a garden, full of color and life."*
REBEL VEGAN

THE REBEL VEGAN PHILOSOPHY

The Vegan Society's official definition of "vegan" is:

> *"... a philosophy and way of living which seeks to exclude - as far as is possible and practicable - all form of exploitation of, and cruelty to, animals for food, clothing, or any other purpose; and by extension, promotes the development and use of animal-free alternatives for the benefit of animals, humans, and the environment."*

For many, this definition might seem intimidating–it's a lot to take on at once. This is why you meet so many naysayers, ex-vegans, and ex-vegetarians. Veganism has been portrayed as an extreme diet, but take a closer look at the definition and you'll see that it accounts for individual circumstances and offers some flexibility.

And put succinctly, veganism is simply a cruelty-free philosophy and way of living. This should not be hijacked by the media and made into an ascetic cult or joke. If you tell yourself that starting tomorrow you will never have cake, cookies, fast food, you will likely cave in rather quickly. The same happens with veganism. I have known vegans who seemed to have had a sudden enlightenment and went from carnism to veganism overnight., But not everyone can nor should. We all have our own paths, even when we share the same goals and ultimate destination.

I recognize that there is not one single way to go vegan. I see veganism as a way to navigate through life, trying to do the best for you and the world. You might go fully vegan, or you might start as a flexitarian. There is a dietary spectrum when it comes to cruelty-free eating, and we are all on it.

While the optimum place for yourself, others, and the planet is veganism, it is true that every step is just that–a step in the right direction. You can work your way along the spectrum at your own speed, using it as a guide for progression, rather than restrictive rules.

	Flexitarianism		Ovo-lacto-vegetarianism		Ovo-vegetarianism	
Carnism		Pescatarianism		Lacto-vegetarianism		Veganism (or plant-based)

The *REBEL VEGAN LIFE* series is to inform and empower readers to make their own decisions about where they fit on the spectrum and what shifts they would like to make in their lives towards a more compassionate way of being.

As your confidence grows, you will gradually move further along the spectrum. I am a realist, and I know that we won't change the current food system and turn the world vegan overnight. This is a long-haul process and transformation of the dominant culture. But we can all be part of this cultural shift and the momentum that this movement is building. By taking this journey, you are a *REBEL VEGAN* and making a positive difference in the world on a daily basis.

This lifestyle is a means to emanate dignity, celebrate life, show compassion, and promote justice. Ultimately, it should not be radical to uphold these values and live a cruelty-free life. I vow to speak the truth, debunk the myths, and uncomplicate the real issues in this heated debate, so that you feel fully empowered and inspired to build your best life.

I believe veganism is the future. After everything we've lived through, and with all the challenges we face globally, it is time for a compassionate revolution. And going vegan is an integral part of that. It may not solve all the problems facing the world, but no solution is complete without it. I know that future generations will remember *REBEL VEGANS* as trailblazers, heralding the changes needed to build a brave new world.

And while this is an urgent and important undertaking, it can also be fun. It is a quest to find new ways to do things. It is a dare to experiment with new recipes and an excuse to taste new flavors. It is the joy you feel when you know you are doing the right thing, and the sense of contentment when your ethics are aligned with your actions. And there is a sense of belonging to a bigger cause and community who are fighting on the right side of history.

This book is your roadmap for this brave new world.

"With this book, I hope to make veganism accessible to everyone. To me, veganism is everyone's to share. It belongs to anyone with compassion and a sense of justice. It's like this book—everybody who finds their way here will take away different things."
REBEL VEGAN

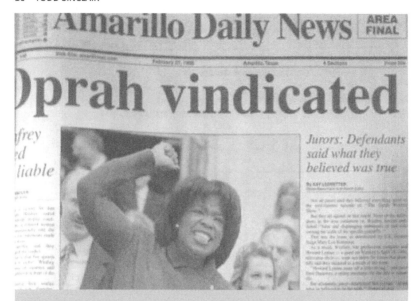

THE MAD COWBOY:
OPRAH'S DAIRY FARMER TURNED VEGAN ACTIVIST

I vividly remember the controversial story that first appeared on the Oprah show about twenty-five years ago. The dormant baby vegan in me was glued to the TV set. It stopped me in my tracks because I knew his story could be my story. The gentle farmer at the center of the storm could have been one of my uncles working the family farm.

Oprah's 'mad cowboy' was often portrayed as "radical" or "extreme", and yet everything he said was calm and rational. It struck a chord with me because he challenged everything I held true at the time, yet also made a lot of sense.

Howard Lyman was a fourth-generation dairy farmer and owned one of the biggest cattle farms in the Midwest. He hit the headlines in 1996 when he challenged America's powerful meat industry on Oprah's show "Dangerous Foods: Could It Happen Here?", where he discussed the possibility of mad cow disease happening in the US, and famously getting Oprah to utter the words "That just stops me cold: I'll never eat another burger."

Oprah was subsequently sued by the Texas cattle industry for $10 million in damages. Although she was eventually victorious, it took two years of litigation whereby she had to relocate her entire show to Texas and to this day seldom speaks on the subject. The actual show has never aired again and can't be found on Youtube. It did make a star of Dr. Phil who was actually Oprah's junior trial lawyer. For most people it highlighted just how sensitive the farming industry is about protecting it's image and position.

Overweight and suffering from sky-high blood pressure, Howard went vegetarian in 1990 and experienced a complete turnaround in his health. A year later, he went vegan and turned his entire life and livelihood upside down. He transformed his factory farm into a wildlife sanctuary, and has been advocating for veganism, organic farming, and animal rights ever since. At 83, Howard is still active in the vegan movement and inspires each new generation.

"I realized my livelihood was built on sand. Everything I'd believed in my entire life was at risk because there I was with a business built on killing animals."
HOWARD LYMAN

I was much too naive to completely understand what Howard was saying, or to challenge my own inbuilt cognitive dissonance to see past my own conditioning. But I also felt he was a trailblazer and truth-speaker. He seemed so solid, just like my uncles, and yet he challenged the status quo and my upbringing. He was the first REBEL VEGAN in my life–someone who made me question the system and want to find out the truth.[1]

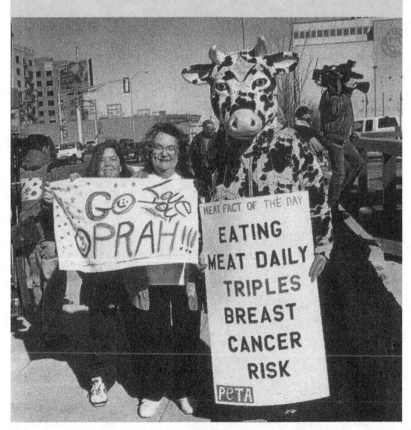

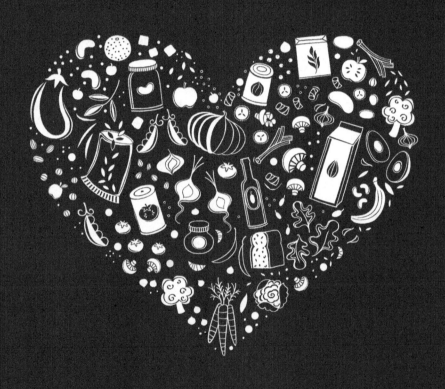

1

A COMPASSIONATE REVOLUTION

"I do not see any reason why animals should be slaughtered to serve as human diet when there are so many substitutes. After all, man can live without meat. Compassion is the radicalism of our time."
THE DALAI LAMA.[1]

What is the core of veganism? There is a lot to it, and we will touch on that soon. But for now, let's keep it simple. Let's start with what veganism is not.

Veganism is not cruel, avoidant, carnistic, nor violent. The modern vegan movement is not some ascetic cult or extreme belief system. It is a philosophy based on kindness and justice for the planet, our fellow earthlings, and ourselves. I believe vegan values are all our shared values. However, veganism is not perfect or some badge of honor that gives free rein to criticize others - whether vegan or not. Veganism doesn't foster callousness nor hostility - quite the opposite, actually. At the core of veganism is compassion. It is an antidote and a reaction to the injustice, lies, and brutality of today's meat industry. Because of this unchecked and corrupted food system, our compassionate revolution has never been so critical, timely, and urgently needed to help solve many issues facing humanity.

Today's industrial global meat industry doesn't consider or protect values like compassion, respect, or truth. As one of history's most powerful industries, it has money as its driving force - profit over welfare and revenue over compassion.

Worryingly, the meat industry's power extends beyond the beings caged in its factories. The industry hurts the animals, the environment, and you without so much as a moment's thought. They have instilled in our society a system of normalized violence based on death, disease, and destruction, and they have called it progress. It is time to rebel, but we need to use an opposite force. Our secret weapons are compassion and justice. My motto is: Knowledge is power. And power should be used with compassion.

WHY A REVOLUTION?

History shows us that the people who end up changing the world - the revolutionaries - are always nuts, until they are right, and then they are geniuses.
JOHN ELIOT[2]

Animal agriculture is the leading cause of species extinction, ocean dead zones, water pollution, and habitat destruction. Livestock and their byproducts account for at least 32,000-million tons of carbon dioxide (CO_2) per year, or 51% of worldwide greenhouse gas emissions. Even without fossil fuels, we will exceed our 565-gigatons CO_2 limit by 2030 - just by raising animals. In addition, 1,100 land activists have been killed in the last twenty years. And this statistic accounts only for the brave people taking a stand in Brazil. And to top it all off, 82% of starving children live in countries where food is fed to livestock instead of to their people, and then the animals are shipped off and eaten by wealthier western countries, leaving the children to starve.[3]

How has humankind let this happen? How have we turned a blind eye to all the suffering and damage? Our food production systems are wreaking havoc on our world, and for what? Profit. Endless greed has allowed the creation and uncontrolled growth of industries that spread pain and suffering and cause waves of extinction around the globe. They don't care about feeding us. If they did, they would take the 135-billion pounds of food fed to cows every day and give some of it to humans who, by the way, only need 21-billion pounds of food per day worldwide.[4] It's time to challenge the systems that have built up around us. What we eat has never mattered more.

It can be hard to grasp how our diets can cause all this harm and destruction. Let's take a closer look at how things have gone wrong.

ANIMAL WELFARE

"We are all animals of this planet. We are all creatures. And non-human animals experience pain sensations just like we do."
JOAQUIN PHOENIX

We are brought up to believe that the consumption of meat, dairy, and eggs is natural, even necessary, to our wellbeing. The image of life on the farm is romanticized until there is no death, gore, or truth left to it in the slightest. You only have to look at children's picture books full of smiling farm animals to appreciate how disconnected we are from reality. I know this moral conflict and cognitive dissonance more than most, having grown up on a dairy farm in eastern Canada.

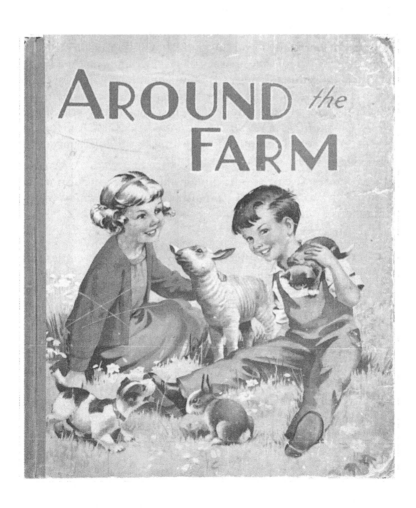

My family loved our animals. My father and his ancestors poured their all into ensuring their care and wellbeing. I grew up seeing the calves as my companions. Our cows were free to graze the fields during the day and slept in warm, comfortable beds of hay in the large wooden barn at night. Our farm was closer to the romanticized image than an industrial farm is, or could ever be. My journey from one end of the diet spectrum to the other has given me perspective. It is only from this distance that I can understand the suffering even in this idealized setting.

Looking back, I can see the pain and torment the animals endured. Even though my family meant well, the practices used at the time still resulted in traumatizing memories of calves crying all night , and the neighbor casually ripping chickens' heads off with his bare hands every time one escaped from their battery cages. I realize now how this was normalized. I was desensitized to the abuse surrounding me.

If my family's humble farm caused harm to the animals they took pride in raising, the harm and terror the animals are experiencing in today's factory farms—where they are seen as product units on an assembly line instead of sentient beings—is unimaginable. If you want to do a deeper dive and gain a true understanding of what is happening on these farms, refer to chapter four of the first book in my series: *REBEL VEGAN A Radical Take in Veganism For a Brave New World*. And for those brave truth seekers, I recommend watching "Earthlings" narrated by Joachin Phoenix (see our Resources section).

But why should we care about animal welfare? We can't bear to see a dog being kicked, yet eat and wear our other fellow animals without a thought.

THIS IS WHY.

Most of us are fully disconnected as to where our food comes from. We brand our meat 'pork' or 'beef', but cringe at the thought of eating 'pig flesh' or 'ground cow'? Have you noticed how the animal agriculture industry shows images of smiling baby animals behind white picket fences at the feet of loving farmers, but never the reality of the horrors of the factory farms? Did you know that many western governments have even introduced legislation to make it illegal for their citizens—us—to take pictures or videos inside farms, where the result of doing so is being placed on the terrorist registry! So damning and alarming is the reality of modern farming methods that they need to build these walls and keep us disconnected.

AND THIS IS WHY.

Animals are conscious, intelligent beings with complex social and emotional needs that cannot be met in a factory farm setting. We know that animals feel pain in the same way that we do; we know they experience emotions just like we do. Studies detailed in National Geographic by evolutionary biologist and author, Marc Bekoff, and postdoctoral fellow at the Natural History Museum of Los Angeles, Bree Putman, tell us that:

> *"Mammals share the same nervous system, neurochemicals, perceptions, and emotions, all of which are integrated into the experience of pain... Reptiles, amphibians, and fish have the neuroanatomy necessary to perceive pain and have been shown to avoid painful stimuli."*[5]

If we really tune into ourselves, we see that we naturally balk at inflicting physical or mental pain onto another creature. More importantly, we know deep down that we don't like the way meat gets on our plate - so much so that we can't even bear to think about it. This is why I believe vegans are often shunned and ridiculed. Our choice to act in line with our innate instincts brings up feelings of cognitive dissonance in those who have chosen to turn away from reality and cling to the status quo of the dominant belief in carnism. That violent ideology that has hoodwinked us all into believing that the Standard Western diet[6] is healthy and natural. My question to those who feel this dissonance, but choose to ignore it and settle for what is on their plate, is this:

If we have to avoid thinking about something to do it, shouldn't that be evidence enough that something is wrong? If you can't bear to view the horrors of what happens inside factory farms, is it right to consume their products and expect nourishment or peace of mind? If any of this disturbs you, it is likely time to nourish the soul and be in alignment with your core values.

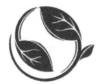

HOW SPECIESISM AND CARNISM ARE UNDERPINNING OUR TREATMENT OF ANIMALS[7]

We only have to compare the value we give to a puppy over a piglet to understand the concept of speciesism. One will lead an indulged life at the heart of our family. The other is considered a product for profit and will be fattened up and slaughtered at six months old, having spent it's brief life in a small pen. Yet there is nothing intrinsic that separates the dog and the pig morally. Scientific studies show that pigs are highly complex animals that can solve puzzles and are actually smarter than dogs. We have created these misguided moral distinctions and this is speciesism.

Speciesism is a form of oppression like racism and is the bias or practice of treating one species as morally more important than other species. I believe our future ancestors will look back at the way we treated and consumed other animals with horror. It is a dark mark on humanity and does not belong in our world. It is a symptom of a society completely disconnected from one simple truth: we are all connected and essential - all of us earthlings, sharing this planet.

"One day the absurdity of the almost universal human belief in the slavery of other animals will be palpable. We shall then have discovered our souls and become worthier of sharing this planet with them."
MARTIN LUTHER KING, JR.

In her groundbreaking book *Why We Love Dogs, Eat Pigs, and Wear Cows: An Introduction to Carnism*, Dr. Melanie Joy first introduced the concept of carnism - the hidden belief system that enables us to support the use and consumption of animal products.

It is based on the assumption that humans have dominion over other animals by divine authority - in other words: animals are merely there to serve humans. Dr. Joy compared carnism to patriarchy, stating that both are dominant ideologies rarely challenged because they are so ubiquitous and yet unspoken.

"We don't see meat-eating as we do vegetarianism, as a choice, based on assumptions about animals, our world and ourselves. Rather, we see it as a given, the 'natural' thing to do, the way things have always been and the way things will always be. We eat animals without thinking about what we are doing and why, because the belief system that underlies this behavior is invisible. This invisible belief system is what I call carnism."

DR. MELANIE JOY[8]

If you have picked up this book, you may already appreciate or empathize that our treatment of other species is somehow intrinsically wrong. You have recognized that there is a disconnect— what I call moral schizophrenia. Maybe you recognize your own cognitive dissonance or unease with your involvement in this violent but unspoken carnist system. This can be a disturbing awakening, as it goes against our conditioning, and everything we have been told is normal and natural. But through discomfort, we grow and evolve. Your move towards a cruelty-free life is part of that evolution. As a *REBEL VEGAN* it's our duty to challenge oppression and fight for justice and compassion.

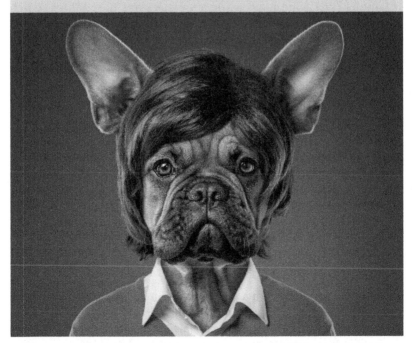

THE ENVIRONMENT: INCONVENIENT SCIENCE

"We must change our diet.
The Planet can't support billions of meat-eaters."
SIR DAVID ATTENBOURGH[9]

Our current food system is simply not sustainable. Not because we can't produce enough food, as we learned above. Our food system is not sustainable because it literally consumes all our resources while destroying the planet we live on. Humanity's taste for flesh will make our children homeless. Animal agriculture is a main driver responsible for speeding up climate change. This is not a statement made up by Peta or a one-off environmental warrior. Eminent climate scientists have been sounding the alarm for decades. Their research shows that the most impactful thing we can do to halt the climate crisis is to reduce our reliance on animal products.[10]

While the greenhouse gas effect can be natural and beneficial, the fact is that the speed at which we increase the concentration of these gases in our atmosphere is causing Earth's temperature to rise. The result is the climate disasters we are witnessing today. Cyclones devastated countries across southern Africa in 2019. At the same time, floods and landslides forced 12-million people from their homes in India, Nepal, and Bangladesh. Australia had the worst bushfire season on record in 2020. Hurricane after hurricane has swept through the southeastern United States, including the infamous Hurricane Ida,[11] while a vicious cycle of wildfires scorch the west.[12] And while it seems like water is an infinitely renewable resource, it's not. Droughts are leaving Central America's Dry Corridor without a successful crop season for the sixth year in a row, and the United Nations has announced that civilization will run out of freshwater by 2050 if we continue to waste this precious resource on animal agriculture. [13] [14]

The industry does not just waste water, it pollutes it beyond repair. Waste from the 70-billion animals raised in factory farms for slaughter each year,[15] consisting of antibiotic-resistant bacteria, hormones, bedding waste, antibiotic residues, chemicals, ammonia, nitrogen, heavy metals, and even dead animals, it runs off into our streams, rivers, and eventually our oceans. The result is ocean dead zones empty of their usual biodiversity. These zones also pose a risk to human health due to the toxic effects of red tides.[16] But why should we care about the biodiversity in the ocean?

In short, if the ocean dies... we die.

The ocean generates fifty percent of the oxygen we breathe. It helps regulate our climate, and it is the driving force of the global circulation system of water between land, sea, and the atmosphere. [17]

OUR HEALTH: LIES THE MEAT INDUSTRY TELLS US

"Everything in food works together
to create health or disease."
T. COLIN CAMPBELL OF THE CHINA STUDY[18]

Meat and dairy have been promoted as the pinnacles of a healthy diet and integral to our survival since the establishment of commercial food production systems. But the truth is we have all been misled and lied to. These foods aren't healthy - in fact, they are dangerous. They give us cancer, heart disease, obesity, and diabetes.[19] My mother taught me the truism that you are what you eat. Every time you eat, you either feed disease or fight it. You can consume vitality and health, or you can consume death or disease. Here I am reminded of the George Bernard Shaw quote: "I choose not to make a graveyard of my body for the rotting corpses of dead animals."[20]

Food is much more than simply fuel. There is truth in the old maxim that food is medicine, as it can either promote or worsen your health. It all depends on what you eat. Meat and dairy have been proven time and time again to cause inflammation, disease, and even death.[21] A plant-based diet of whole foods has been shown to not only prevent many chronic diseases, but may help treat some conditions, such as type 2 diabetes. Increasingly, the diet commonly prescribed to prevent, treat, and even reverse these diseases is a plant-based diet.

ANTIBIOTIC RESISTANCE: OUR FUTURE HEALTH UNDER THREAT
Meat and dairy also lead to antibiotic resistance. The Antimicrobial Resistance Global Report released by the World Health Organisation (WHO) states that antimicrobial resistance is a:

"...widespread serious threat [that] is no longer a prediction for the future, it is happening right now in every region of the world and has the potential to affect anyone, of any age, in any country."[22]

It is widespread and even necessary to misuse huge quantities of antibiotics on livestock, just so they can survive the brutal conditions of factory farming. It is estimated that worldwide 73% of all antibiotics are used on farm animals, not people. It became routine, as it enabled the animals to be kept in such appalling and unnatural conditions where disease would normally spread quickly. Even though the FDA banned the use of medically important antibiotics as growth promoters, the quantity of antibiotics sold for food-producing animals has been on the rise.[23] As a result, we are seeing an increase of antibiotic-resistant superbugs. Even our most commonplace and vital antibiotics, such as penicillin, are becoming obsolete. Without a massive shift in how we farm and produce food, we are heading towards another international health crisis.

The UK Government carried out an extensive study in 2019 and found that if we don't make changes to current farming practices, the number of deaths per year could increase to 10 million per year by 2050 - this would surpass the total deaths annually from cancer. This also has huge financial implications - with a cumulative cost of 11 trillion dollars. The World Bank estimates this would force 28 million people into extreme poverty.[24]

THE SOCIAL FACTOR:

"If you have men who will exclude any of God's creatures from the shelter of compassion and pity, you will have men who will deal likewise with their fellow men."
ST FRANCIS OF ASSISI[25]

"At his best, man is the noblest of all animals; separated from law and justice he is the worst."
ARISTOTLE[26]

This is the least known reason for changing your diet and to rebel against the current food system. However, as little as we recognize it, meat production heavily influences our culture and how society functions. For instance, the animal agriculture industry is one of the factors leading to social inequality. The industry provides jobs, but the treatment of their employees is comparable to modern-day slavery. The work is traumatizing, exploitative, hazardous, and grossly underpaid. And who is the industry giving these jobs to? Often it is destitute, the poor, and the illegal immigrants who have no voice, access to health care, and opportunities for advancement. They are stuck in this exploitative system.

People living near the slaughterhouses and factory farms are involuntarily suffering for our food choices as well. They have to endure air polluted with neurotoxins and chemicals that lead to respiratory conditions and even particles of feces. [27] The undesirable living conditions created by these factory operations often leads to them being located in impoverished communities where the people don't have the resources to fight back. They can't afford to fight, they can't afford to leave, and they certainly can't afford to treat the health burdens being forced upon them and their families.

If you care about equality and justice, then you care about vegan values.

COVID AND VEGANISM:

"What we eat matters all the more now."
BRITISH MEDICAL JOURNAL

It might be hard to see it at first, but COVID has put veganism on the map. It has exposed the old systems as dangerous and highlighted the urgent need for vegan values. And once you can see it, you can't unsee it.

Restaurants closing down and grocery stores facing scarcity of products allowed us the opportunity to pause, reflect, and prepare for what is being called the 'new normal'. More and more of us realize that we don't want to go back to our unsustainable or unhealthy ways, the effects of which are more prominent now than ever. We recognize that we need to move forward in a more mindful way, so we can avoid this happening again.

COVID has highlighted how essential our diet is in shaping our health. The brutal statistics have shown that people with high blood pressure, heart disease, diabetes, and obesity have a much higher risk of COVID-related mortality. We know that our standard Western diet is a huge factor in the development of these diseases. We also know that whole food, plant-based diets reduce the risk of all these health conditions, meaning changing the way we eat has never been more critical.

Beyond recognizing the seriousness of the health crises facing both ourselves and our planet, we recognized the need to not only prepare for future pandemics, but also to prevent them. Ending the exploitation of animals, and our intimate interaction with wildlife and mistreated factory-farmed animals through a plant-based lifestyle, is one of the biggest actions we can take to protect ourselves against future pandemics.

Animals in factory farms, backyard farms, and wildlife markets are held in horrifying conditions. Investigators from The Independent found animals living in pens with corpses in an advanced state of putrefaction, and containers overflowing with animal corpses covered in larvae. These are not isolated incidents, but a normal part of these operations. These conditions lead to the transmission of viruses between different species and humans, and could lead to another covid-like pandemic.[28]

Three out of four emerging infectious diseases come from animals. Every pandemic in recorded human history has come from our mistreatment of animals. Fifty-six zoonotic diseases are responsible for an estimated 2.5-billion cases of human illness, and 2.7-million deaths per year.[29] We have been relatively fortunate that covid wasn't more infectious or deadly.

This has given us a critical window of opportunity to rethink our food production and change our behavior. We need to learn these hard lessons. If we do not, the next pandemic could be much worse. And without a fundamental shift in the treatment of animals, it is not a question of if, but when.

If we want to protect our health, both individual and global, we must shift towards a diet that supports our immune systems while reducing the pressure on the planet. I often say that the problem is on our plate. Luckily, so is the solution.

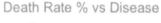

Death Rate % vs Disease

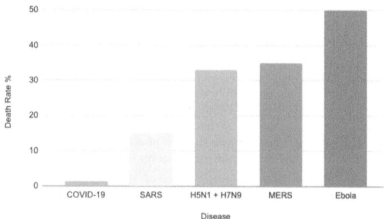

WHERE DO WE START?

With the science and warnings piling up, it becomes obvious that our diets and relationship with meat must change. It is the only way to protect our future. If you're anything like me, by now the voice in your head is probably screaming:

"But what can I do?"

I know I felt this way when I first learned the truth about the animal industry. I was enraged. I felt misled and disrespected. I wanted nothing to do with a system based on violence and inequality. It was time to rebel and fight for this brave new world.

We can protest, we can educate, we can fight through legislation - and we should. But there is something every person can do every day. Each day, you can save 1,100 gallons of water, forty-five pounds of grain, thirty square feet of forested land - working to clean our air and regulate the Earth's temperature, twenty pounds of CO_2 equivalent, and one animal's life.... Simply by choosing compassion, simply by going vegan. [30]

REBEL VEGAN wants to start a compassionate revolution and forge a new, respectful relationship with other animals, with the planet, and among our fellow humans too. Throughout the pages of this book, I will help you take steps towards positive change. I aim to give you everything you need to start your new, compassionate, revolutionary life.

GET READY TO VEGANIZE YOUR WORLD ONE STEP AT A TIME.

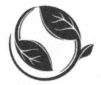

2

VEGANOMETRY
PLANT-BASED HEALTH HANDBOOK

"The beef industry has contributed to more American deaths than all the wars of this century, all natural disasters, and all auto-mobile accidents combined. If beef is your idea of 'real food for real people' you'd better live real close to a real good hospital."
DR. NEAL D. BARNARD[1]

"The most ethical diet just so happens to be the most environmentally sound diet and just so happens to be the healthiest."
DR. MICHAEL GREGER[2]

Fasten your seatbelts. This may shock you, it may disturb you, but it turns the long-accepted diet model on its head. According to medical scientists from Harvard University, the optimum amount of meat for a healthy diet is...precisely zero.[3]

The science regarding our current diet is in. It is overwhelming, consistent, and conclusive. The leading cause for premature death and disability in the United States is the standard American (or Western) diet.[4] This sobering statistic was the result of the largest ever study of risk factors for disease (the Global Burden of Disease Study), which examined deaths and their causes between 1990 and 2016.[5]

While it makes sombre reading–after all, the study concludes that we've been making ourselves sick with every bite–it also offers hope. Because if our current way of eating has the power to make us unwell, then it also has the power to heal. If we veganize our diet, we can live longer, healthier lives...as well as be kinder to the environment and animals.

For your shift towards veganism to be successful, you need the tools and information to support your decision and a new way of life. If you're currently eating the standard Western diet–in which your meals are based around meat, dairy and eggs–simply removing animal products from your plate will likely leave you without enough calories or nutrients.

This is why many people who attempt a vegan diet return to eating meat, quoting tiredness and hunger as the main reasons. An understanding of what makes a healthy, balanced, plant-based diet will help you give your body everything it needs to thrive. This chapter will give you that information so that you can begin to sustainably and successfully transition to a plant-based diet.

One of the oldest arguments leveled against veganism is the threat of malnourishment. The stereotype of the pale, thin vegan joylessly eating kale, lentils and brown rice for eternity is still present in many minds. The first question you've probably been asked if you've told anyone you're going plant-based is "but where will you get your protein/calcium/B12?"

Funny isn't it, how everyone becomes an expert, and people who have previously been unconcerned about any aspect of your diet suddenly become nutritionists when they find out you're going vegan. Well, fear not! You can find all the nutrients your body needs in plants! And once you've finished reading this, you will be able to debunk many of the vegan nutrition myths that may be thrown your way.

Before we begin, I just want to explore and demystify the magical quality that seems to surround meat and dairy. Then, we'll get into the macro and micro-nutrients you need for health, and where you can find them. Plus, we'll see how veganism can help you get to your ideal weight without counting calories (most of us have put on a little weight since Covid hit, and now it's time to shed those pounds!).

WHY IS MEAT PROMOTED AS PART OF A HEALTHY DIET?

"Collectively the media; the meat, oil, and dairy industries; and our own government are not presenting accurate advice about the healthiest way to eat."

DR. CALDWELL ESSELSTYN[6]

If the science is in, telling us that plant-based nutrition is the healthiest option while meat and dairy contribute to disease, then why is there still such a strong reaction and skepticism around this topic? It turns out that this confusion is by design rather than by accident.

This is not the first time that powerful industries have attempted to pull the wool over our eyes. Fifty years ago, the tobacco industry used athletes, doctors, and soldiers as spokespeople to promote their products. Some of their adverts were even aimed at pregnant women (like Nico Time Cigarettes: "The smooth taste expectant mothers crave"). Among the claims were promises that smoking could calm an irritated throat, lessen coughing, and improve appetite management.[7]

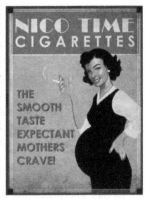

When the harmful consequences of smoking began getting known, the tobacco industry funded its own studies to disprove any negative effects, while "proving" that smoking didn't actually cause cancer.[8] These days, we would laugh if anyone tried telling us smoking is good for the body. The tide is turning on our diets too.

The industrial farming industry, large food corporations, and fast-food retailers use the same strategies as the tobacco industry did for decades to confuse the public about the dangers of their products. Backed by billions of dollars in profit and government subsidies, these industries are able to fund misleading studies, influence politicians, use celebrities to endorse their products, and put out clever marketing campaigns designed to keep the masses misinformed. What's more, their close ties to governments means certain foods remain on national nutritional guidelines, even though independent studies demonstrate that these foods cause disease and premature death.

I will give one example to illustrate this, but if you'd like to delve deeper into the murky world of industrial farming subsidies and corruption, head to Chapter 3 of my companion book, *REBEL VEGAN LIFE: A Radical New Take On Veganism For A Brave New World.*

In 2015, the World Health Organization (WHO) and International Agency for Research on Cancer (IARC) published a report on meat and cancer. They examined over 800 epidemiological studies and concluded that consuming meat poses a carcinogenic threat to humans. So much so that red meat was classified as a Group 2A carcinogen ("probably carcinogenic to humans") and processed meat as a Group 1 carcinogen ("carcinogenic to humans").[9] For comparison, tobacco and asbestos are both Group 1 carcinogens. Now, you might expect governments to take this information and act accordingly, for example, by publishing nutrition guidelines that help people reduce their consumption of animal products.

Another logical strategy would be to no longer advertise meat and dairy, or to put health warnings on fast food packaging, as they have done with cigarettes. Nothing of the sort has happened. In fact, US nutrition guidelines have remained largely unchanged for 15 years and still recommend a daily intake of meat and dairy.[10]

Clearly, it is up to us to do the research, question the status quo, and make the changes to create a just and sustainable future. That's what being a *REBEL VEGAN* is all about.

THE DANGERS OF MEAT, DAIRY AND SEAFOOD

"The most ethical diet just so happens to be the most environmentally sound diet and just so happens to be the healthiest."
DR. MICHAEL GREGER[11]

The accepted narrative and ingrained belief system are that animal products are essential for athletic muscles, strong bones, and a healthy brain. But while meat and dairy are promoted as health-boosting foods, the reality is they aren't. Yes, they contain protein, B12, and heme iron, but they also contain saturated fat, cholesterol, and chemical residues from animal medications and animal feed.

These increase the risk of chronic non-communicable diseases, such as heart disease and cancer. Non-communicable diseases are lifestyle-related–our lifestyle is the number one killer. Often with little thought, we are making these potentially dangerous and important choices at every meal.

Here is a quick and dirty review of why meat, dairy, and even fish don't need to feature on your plate.

- Red and processed meat contain nitrates, saturated fat and other chemicals that increase the risk of colorectal cancer by 24%.[12] They also significantly increase the risk of cardiovascular disease, heart attacks and strokes.[13]
- Fish contain environmental pollutants such as methyl-mercury, polychlorinated biphenyls and mercury, which increase the risk of cardiovascular disease[14] and cognitive decline.[15]
- The FDA recommends that women of childbearing age should avoid fish because of mercury poisoning (a shockingly telling warning as far as I'm concerned!).[16]
- Dairy contains IGF-1 (insulin-like growth factor 1), which has been associated with an increased risk of cancer, diabetes, and chronic inflammation.[17]
- Dairy increases the risk of breast cancer by up to 80%.[18]
- Dairy increases the risk of prostate cancer by up to 65%.[19]
- Long-term consumption of eggs clogs the arteries and causes as much damage to blood vessels as smoking[20] (it is now illegal for egg manufacturers to advertise eggs as nutritious.[21])

CARDIOVASCULAR DISEASES:
Heart Diseases, Stroke, Heart Attack, Aorta Disease, Deep Vein Thrombosis.

Cardiovascular diseases are the leading cause of mortality globally, causing 32% of all deaths. Around 18 million people die because of heart disease (heart attacks and strokes) every year.[22]

Cardiovascular disease is caused by a build-up of fatty deposits (or plaque) in the blood vessels, which stop blood from flowing as it should to the brain or to the heart. One of the principal factors is diet–an excess of saturated fat and refined sugars, basically the two mainstays of the standard Western diet.

Diet is the cause of cardiovascular disease, and it can also be the antidote. A review of studies published in the journal *Trends in Cardiovascular Medicine* states that plant-based diets should be recommended as an environmentally sustainable dietary option to improve cardiovascular health.[23]

CANCER
Cancer is the second leading cause of death, causing 9.6 million deaths every year, or 1 in 6 deaths.[24]

It happens when normal cells begin to malfunction and mutate into tumors. While many still think that cancer is something that happens by accident or because of defective genes, the truth is that our lifestyle is mostly to blame.

According to a new study by the American Institute for Cancer Research, 42% of cancers are linked to risk factors we can control: excess weight, poor diet, and lack of physical activity.[25] Observational studies show that plant-based diets can reduce the risk of cancer by at least 10-12%.[26] Their protective effects come from the fiber, antioxidants and vitamins contained in vegetables, fruits, and other whole foods.

OBESITY

Worldwide obesity has almost tripled since 1975. According to the World Health Organization, 2 billion adults are overweight or obese, and at least 2.8 million people die each year as a result.[27] It is increasingly affecting children too - the proportion of obese or overweight 5-19 year olds has quadrupled from 4% in 1975 to 18% in 2016.[28]

Obesity is not a genetic disease. It is caused by an over-consumption of processed foods, low in nutrients, and high in fat and sugar. Ultimately, our current way of eating means that the population of the world's richest nations are simultaneously overfed but undernourished.

When it comes to weight management, shifting away from processed foods and towards whole plant foods is the best thing we can do. This is confirmed by a study published in the American Journal of Lifestyle Medicine, which states: "A diet centered on whole plant foods appears to be a safe, simple, sustainable solution to the obesity epidemic."[29]

TYPE 2 DIABETES

Around the world, 422 million people have diabetes. Tellingly, these are concentrated in wealthy nations with higher meat consumption rates. This disease causes 1.6 million deaths every year.[30]

Diabetes is characterized by high levels of blood sugar, which over time leads to damage to the nerves, blood vessels, eyes, kidneys, and heart. This happens when the body is unable to make enough insulin or becomes resistant to insulin, usually due to an excess intake of sugar. Diabetes is another disease that is both caused by– and preventable through–diet.

A study published in the European Journal of Epidemiology found that compared to meat-heavy diets, plant-based diets lower the risk of insulin resistance, pre-diabetes, and type 2 diabetes.[31]

DEMENTIA AND ALZHEIMER'S DISEASE

Worldwide, 50 million people have dementia, of which Alzheimer's is the most common form. There are around 10 million new cases of dementia each year.[32]

Dementia is a progressive disease that causes a deterioration in memory, thinking, emotional control, behavior, and the ability to live independently. While it mostly affects older people, it is not a normal part of ageing. Studies show that diet-induced chronic inflammation and metabolic changes cause an acceleration of our cognitive decline.[33] Here again, our diet can either exacerbate or prevent this disease.

A study published by the *Journal Innovation in Aging* found that compared to non-vegetarians, people on a plant-based diet had a 38% lower risk of dementia.[34]

COVID-19

At the time of writing, there have been around 254 million cases and 5 million people have died from Covid.[35]

Covid-19 is not a chronic disease, but nonetheless, it has shone a spotlight on global health and the role of our diets. While questions still remain about exactly how the virus became a global pandemic, what we do know is that our ability to survive is in great part linked to our current state of health.

Studies show that people with obesity, diabetes, existing health conditions, or compromised immune systems are more likely to get Covid and to suffer complications. While diet alone cannot guarantee that you will avoid getting sick, a healthy diet does support a strong immune system–and a strong immune system is your body's defense against illness.

The science is clear when it comes to boosting immunity–a plant-based diet is the best solution. Centered around whole grains, beans, pulses, vegetables, fruits, nuts, and seeds, this diet is packed with nutrients that help the body stay healthy. And when your body is thriving, you are less likely to get sick.

In May 2021, a study published in the *British Medical Journal* compared the impact of different diets on Covid severity. Researchers found that plant-based diets and pescatarian diets were associated with a lower risk of moderate-to-severe Covid-19. They concluded that these types of diets can protect against severe Covid-19.[36]

"The beef industry has contributed to more American deaths than all the wars of this century, all natural disasters, and all automobile accidents combined.
If beef is your idea of 'real food for real people,' you'd better live real close to a real good hospital."
NEAL D. BARNARD MD,
AUTHOR OF FOODS THAT FIGHT PAIN.[37]

IS JUST GOING VEGAN THE ANSWER?

Not entirely. And that's why it's so important to understand what makes a healthy diet. With big food producers bringing out vegan products, you can easily be a junk food vegan these days. And while this means you're not directly contributing to animal cruelty, it doesn't necessarily mean you're doing the best for your body.

Veganism is rooted in compassion–compassion for the animals, the planet, and fellow humans–and it's about trying your best to avoid inflicting harm. I think this should be extended to ourselves as well, and that means choosing foods that support the body rather than damage it.

The standard Western diet is characterized by a high intake of meat and dairy, but also a lot of sugar and processed foods–these foods harm the body. Plant-based foods, on the other hand, support health and longevity.

THE PROBLEM WITH SUGAR:
INFLAMMATION, OBESITY AND DIABETES

"History has demonstrated that a diet of specific vegan foods, eaten in a specific caloric ratio, will meet all our criteria. For healing inflammatory bowel diseases, other gut disorders and most other illnesses, I have learned which are the most beneficial foods of all. Those foods comprise what I call the Vegan Healing Diet."
DR. DAVID KLEIN[38]

We are consuming way too much sugar, and it is making us both fat and sick. Americans eat an average of 126g (30 teaspoons) of sugar a day.[39] The recommended intake according to the latest US nutritional guidelines is no more than 50 grams (12 teaspoons).[40] According to other health institutions, such as the NHS (the UK's National Health Service), this should be no more than 30 grams (7.25 teaspoons).[41] We are far from this ideal. Taking this into account, it is no wonder we suffer from so many preventable health problems.

There are two main ways that sugar damages your health. The first has to do with oxidative stress and inflammation. The second has to do with weight gain and diabetes.

Researchers have observed that excess sugar triggers a spike in free radicals.[42] Free radicals are chemicals that come from pollution and other toxins; they are also formed as by-products of your cells normal functioning (a little bit like exhaust fumes are a by-product of driving a car).

When there are too many free radicals circulating in the body, they cause something called oxidative stress. This process damages cell membranes, as well as causing DNA mutations that can trigger chronic disease.[43] Oxidative stress is one of the main factors in premature ageing. Free radicals also increase inflammation in the body, and this increases your risk of chronic diseases (we'll look at inflammation in a moment).

When it comes to weight gain and diabetes, this has to do with how sugar is metabolized by the body. When you eat carbohydrates, your body breaks them down into glucose, which your cells can use as fuel. When glucose hits your bloodstream, your pancreas releases insulin–this is a hormone that signals to your cells to absorb the glucose.

When you eat too many carbohydrates or foods that contain a lot of sugar (such as processed foods and fizzy drinks), your pancreas has to pump out more and more insulin to try to get the glucose out of your bloodstream and into your cells. Over time, cells stop responding to the insulin–this is known as insulin resistance, which is the first step towards type 2 diabetes.

The other problem with insulin is that it also signals to the body to store any excess glucose as either glycogen (this is stored in your liver as readily available energy) or as fat (this happens when your glycogen stores are full). This is how sugar, which is technically fat-free (and, ironically, added to many no-fat or low-fat diet foods), actually causes excess body fat.

THE PROBLEM WITH PROCESSED FOODS:
CONVENIENT FOR YOUR SCHEDULE, NOT YOUR BODY

Processed foods are the ready-made foods we grab because it's convenient. According to a study by the British Medical Journal, over half of Americans' calories come from ultra-processed foods.[44] These are foods that have been taken apart and then put together again with added sweeteners, salt, oils, artificial additives and preservatives.

It wasn't that long ago that most people ate real food that was cooked at home from natural ingredients. These days, we just pick up something ready-made because it's faster. I mean, who has time to cook anyway? Programs like MasterChef have made us a little wary of stepping into the kitchen; we worry that cooking is a complex procedure that involves fidgety recipes, expensive gadgets, and hard-to-find ingredients. Ready-made meals are so much more convenient. But they are not convenient for our bodies.

As an example, let's take the average loaf of supermarket bread. It is made with a complex mix of refined flours, sugar, emulsifiers, preservatives, synthetic vitamins (which have to be added back in because the refining process strips the grains of their nutrients), and even dehydrated milk! On the other hand, homemade bread (or freshly made bread from a good bakery) contains whole grain flour, natural yeast, and water. The two will have a dramatically different impact on the body.

Processed food is any food that has been subjected to cleaning, heating, milling, chopping, pasteurizing, blanching, cooking, freezing, drying, dehydrating, mixing, packaging, or any other procedure that alters the original food source from its natural states, such as the addition of preservatives, flavorings, colors or other substances approved for use in food products.

I know what you're thinking–doesn't that mean most foods are processed? In a way, yes. We "process" foods when we cook them. So in effect, not all processed foods are bad – in fact, some are very handy to have in your kitchen because they make plant-based eating easier, such as canned beans.

Processed foods range from minimally processed to heavily processed:

- Minimally processed foods: such as roasted nuts, bagged salad, pre-chopped vegetables. These tend not to contain any additives.
- Foods processed to lock in nutritional value and freshness: such as canned tomatoes, canned vegetables and beans, plant milks, or frozen fruits and vegetables. Most of these do not contain added preservatives or ingredients (but you have to check the label, because some, particularly non-organic ones, contain added sugar, preservatives, and even artificial colors).
- Foods with added ingredients (like sugar, salt, oils, colors or preservatives) for flavor or texture: such as pasta sauces, salad dressings, cake mixes, sweetened yogurts, supermarket bread, sauces, dip, cheese slices, hot dogs, and processed meat products (like chicken nuggets).
- Ready to eat foods (these are the most heavily processed foods): such as crackers, biscuits, deli meats, crisps/chips, frozen ready-meals, microwaveable dinners, fizzy drinks, chilled desserts, sweets, candy.

When I say that processed foods should be avoided, I don't mean that you have to start preparing everything from scratch. Minimally processed foods (the first two bullet points) have a place in a healthy, balanced diet. For example, plant milk, frozen fruits and vegetables, roasted nuts and seeds, and canned beans do not have to be avoided. They contain nutrients that support health and help you move towards a vegan diet, while ensuring you give your body everything it needs.

So which processed foods should you avoid? They are easy to recognize. They tend to have a long shelf-life, and their ingredient label reads like a science experiment. They contain ingredients that sound like nothing you would have in your cupboards, such as:

- Monosodium glutamate: added to increase a food's umami flavor and to stimulate appetite. This additive has been linked to neurological issues and metabolic syndrome.[45]
- Erythrosine: added to make foods red. This additive has been linked to thyroid tumors.[46]
- Sodium nitrate: added to make processed meats salty and pink in color. This additive could increase the risk of stomach cancer.[47]
- Carrageenan: added as a thickener and preservative. This additive can trigger inflammation and digestive problems.[48]
- Sodium benzoate: added as a preservative, often found in fizzy drinks. This additive has been linked to ADHD[49] and cancer.[50]

As you can see, these ingredients are added to increase shelf life and to stimulate our taste buds so that we want to buy the product again (this is known in the industry as "repeat appeal"). Health and nutrition have little to do with it; it's more about profits and market share.

Another problem with ultra-processed foods is that they are empty calories. Empty, because they are devoid of nutrients. In other words, they do not contain the essential vitamins and minerals we need for optimum health. They just provide poor quality fuel (usually in the form of refined grains, sugars and fats) alongside a portion of chemicals that the body struggles to process and eliminate.

Let's compare a couple more foods, before we move on to the foundations of a healthy diet, and how you can begin to transition towards a way of eating that supports you while supporting animals and the planet.

The average ready-made salad dressing contains rapeseed oil, milk, eggs, sugar, artificial flavors and colors, ingredients that stress the body. On the other hand, you could very quickly throw together a simple salad dressing of olive oil, lemon juice, a pinch of salt, and maybe some parsley or mint - this would provide you with some healthy fats from the olive oil and inflammation-busting antioxidants from the lemon juice and herbs.

You could make a simple, filling meal in under 30 minutes by quickly stir-frying some vegetables and tofu, adding a splash of soy sauce and spoonful of peanut butter, and serve this alongside some buckwheat noodles or brown rice. This meal would provide you with antioxidants and fiber (vegetables), protein (tofu, peanut butter), healthy fats (peanuts) and complex carbohydrates (buckwheat noodles), which would fill you up and nourish you. Or you could buy a ready meal and pop it in the microwave, but because it is packed with sugar and made with refined ingredients, you're likely to feel hungry again within an hour.

Processed foods might look like the quicker, easier option–especially if you have a busy schedule– but they are not the smartest option when it comes to your health. I'm not saying that you must avoid all processed foods. After all, what is life without the occasional indulgence?

But it is about balance. I'm all about the 80-20 rule, which allows for a little deviation from whole foods. That means that most of your diet is made up of whole foods or minimally processed foods, with the occasional indulgence. The aim is not perfection, but to create the kind of diet you can sustain for life AND enjoy.

> *"When adopting a plant-based diet has been scientifically proven not only to stop the evolution of certain diseases, but it can also reverse them, we then have the moral responsibility to act upon and align our beliefs with our actions. Taking the courage to look the elephant in the eye."*
> **HAYEK HOSPITAL GOES PLANT-BASED**[51]

MESSING WITH YOUR IMMUNE SYSTEM

Your immune system is your personal protection mechanism against disease and infection. Like a bodyguard, it patrols the body and destroys any chemicals, germs or parasites that put your health in danger. The immune system is able to recognize the cells that make up your body and eliminate anything unfamiliar or threatening. When you think about it, you are quite vulnerable. After all, we live in a toxic soup of microscopic bacteria, viruses, parasites, and toxins. These land on our skin, they're in the air we breathe, and the foods we eat. We survive thanks to our immune system, which works tirelessly to keep us safe.

This protective action can turn into a problem, for example, if your immune system reacts to something harmless (such as dust or pollen), or if it turns on itself (as is the case in autoimmune conditions). What makes the immune system over-react in this way? Chronic inflammation.

Chronic inflammation is something almost all of us struggle with to some degree, because of the way we live. Stress levels, polluted air, and processed food all cause an inflammatory response. While this response is normal and even desirable, it puts the immune system under stress. And we all know what happens when we become overwhelmed: we begin making mistakes.

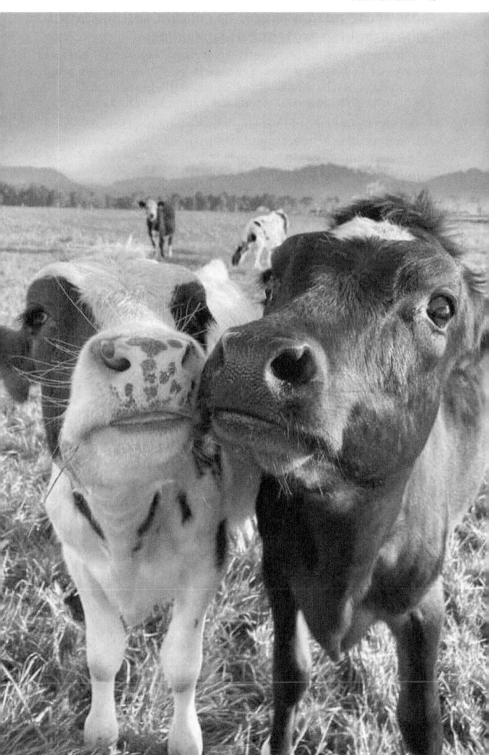

FROM ACUTE INFLAMMATION TO CHRONIC INFLAMMATION - OUR DISRUPTED PROTECTION MECHANISM

Your immune system, or personal bodyguard, has several tools at its disposal to keep you safe. The one it uses most often is acute inflammation. You have no doubt experienced this in your life, if you've ever been bitten by a mosquito, sprained your wrist, or had a cold.

At the first sign of something being amiss—whether that's detecting a foreign substance (insect venom or virus) or damage (like a muscle tear)—your immune system springs into action. The symptoms of acute inflammation are easy to recognize:

- Redness: This is due to increased blood flow as the immune system sends white blood cells to the area.

- Swelling: This happens because of the extra fluids that carry immune cells to the site and carry away dead or damaged cells.

- Heat: Increased blood flow and fluids create more heat in the body.

- Pain: Caused by the by-products of these chemicals stimulating nerve endings.

- Timely: The symptoms last only until they're needed, usually between 2 days and 6 weeks.[52]

- If you have a cold, the symptoms you experience are due to your immune system's acute inflammation response. A red stuffy nose (swelling and redness), a fever (heat), and aching muscles (pain) are all signs that your body is working to get rid of the cold virus.

While acute inflammation is uncomfortable, it is a beneficial and healing process. Once the virus has been eliminated, the insect bite healed, or the muscle recovered, the symptoms disappear.

Chronic inflammation, on the other hand, is not beneficial. It is acute inflammation gone haywire. It happens when your immune system has too much to do. When your personal bodyguard is on constant high alert, it launches its inflammatory response constantly in order to combat substances that shouldn't be in your body.

Certain foods, particularly foods that contain excess sugar and artificial additives (meat, dairy, fish and processed foods, in other words), cause a temporary (acute) inflammatory response. If these foods are eaten regularly, this inflammatory response becomes chronic. When this happens, the effects go from being healing to being damaging.

Chronic inflammation eventually damages healthy cells, tissues and organs, and leads to DNA damage, cellular disfunction and internal scarring. This then sets the scene for many chronic diseases–obesity, diabetes, heart disease, and cancer all have their roots in chronic inflammation.

According to the National Institute of Health, three out of every five deaths are due to diseases caused by chronic inflammation.[53] What's more, chronic inflammation makes it harder for your body to deal with illness or a virus. This is why people with a compromised immune system or those already struggling with inflammatory diseases are at higher risk of getting Covid or dying from it.

Stopping chronic inflammation in its tracks is a vital part of staying healthy and preventing disease. In order to do this, we must move away from the foods that cause inflammation, and move towards foods that actively fight inflammation and give the immune system what it needs to keep working effectively. We must transition to a diet that supports health.

What kind of diet is that? A whole-foods, plant-based diet. It's easier than you might think, once you know the foundations of a healthy, balanced diet. In the next chapter, we master the basics of a nutritious diet. Let's veganize our lives!

VEGAN DIET APPROPRIATE FOR ALL STAGES OF LIFE

The Canadian Dietetic Association, Dietitians of Canada, the British Dietetic Association and the American Dietetic Association have all come out in support of a vegan diet.

According to these recognized and respected institutions:

"Well planned vegan and other types of vegetarian diets are appropriate for all stages of the life cycle, including during pregnancy, lactation, infancy, childhood and adolescence." They go on to say that plant-based diets offer:

"a number of nutritional benefits, including lower levels of saturated fats, cholesterol, and animal protein, as well as higher levels of carbohydrates, fiber, magnesium, potassium, folate, and antioxidants such as vitamins C and E and phytochemicals."[54]

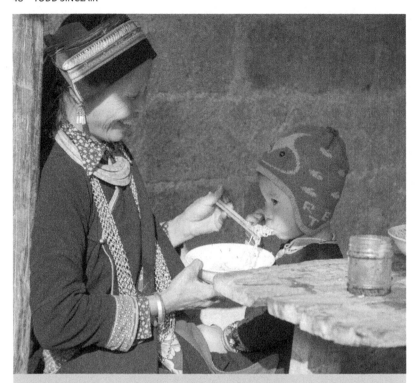

THE CHINA STUDY: NO TURNING BACK FOR VEGANISM[55]

We have known for decades that a plant-based diet holds the key to our health and longevity. In 1998, the China study hit the headlines with groundbreaking findings: our standard Western diet was killing us. The solution was veganism.

In the early 1980s, nutritional biochemist T. Colin Campbell from Cornell University set up a working partnership with the Chinese Academy of Preventative Medicine to study the connection between nutrition and disease. They called it the China Project. China offered a great opportunity to explore this because the population stayed in small areas and communities, and many regions relied on an almost entirely plant-based diet that was both low in fat and high in fiber—the exact opposite to the standard Western diet. This provided a great platform from which to compare the health of rural Chinese and the comparatively rich Americans.

Dr. Campbell was the first to argue for a plant-based diet. His 20-year study looked at mortality rates from cancer and other chronic diseases in 65 counties in China, and found that the consumption of animal products and dairy increases the risk of chronic illnesses, such as cardiovascular disease, diabetes, breast cancer, prostate cancer, and bowel cancer.

Still today, this is considered one of the most comprehensive studies on nutrition ever carried out, and conclusively showed the dangers of a diet high in animal products, as well as the protective effect of a whole foods, plant-based diet. What shocked America and the world was how disturbing the comparison was between the health and weight of Chinese and American populations.

One of the study's biggest findings was the difference between how animal protein and plant protein behave in the body. It found that the proteins in animal foods cause both normal cells and cancerous cells to grow.

Animal proteins also trigger the production of growth factors (such as insulin-like growth factors), which increase the risk of cancer. On the other hand, plant proteins protect cells and do not promote cancer. The researchers' big takeaway was that cancer cells can be turned on or off simply by altering your diet and how much meat and casein proteins you eat.

Another important finding was that a whole foods, plant-based diet, does more than just prevent cancer – it is beneficial for a number of other diseases. During his study, Dr. Campbell realized how much the chronic diseases have in common. Because of these commonalities, it makes sense that proper nutrition both prevents disease and improves health. A plant-based diet can never be "bad" for you, only beneficial.

Ultimately, Campbell's book showed the West that it isn't necessary to eat meat. His book had such an impact that Bill Clinton became a vegan after reading it. To this day, the China Study is considered one of the most important studies into the connection between diet and health. There was no turning back!

"Nutrition that is truly beneficial for one chronic disease will support health across the board."
T. COLIN CAMPBELL

"Going vegan has kept me alive."
BILL CLINTON

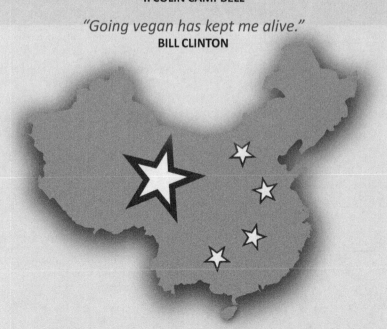

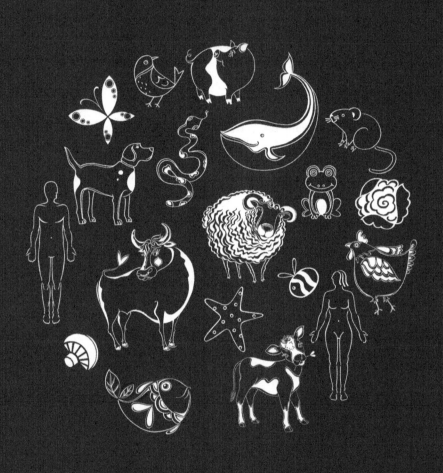

3

COMPLETE NUTRITIONAL
GETTING ALL YOU NEED FROM PLANTS

"People feel poorly because they are nourished by foods you wouldn't feed to your dog and cat. The rich western diet is full of fat, sugar, cholesterol, salt, animal protein — all the wrong foods for people."
DR. JOHN MCDOUGALL[1]

"Food is really and truly the most effective medicine."
DR. JOEL FUHRMAN[2]

THE FOUNDATIONS OF A HEALTHY, BALANCED DIET

For optimum health, the body needs certain macro and micro-nutrients. Macro (meaning "big" in Greek) nutrients are the ones you need in large quantities: complex carbohydrates, protein, and healthy fats. Micro (meaning "small" in Greek) nutrients are those you need in smaller quantities: vitamins, minerals and antioxidants.

In this section, I'm going to break down why each of these nutrients is important for health, and where you can find them. In the next chapter, you'll find a step-by-step guide to begin putting this new knowledge into practice.

PROTEIN

I'll start with this one because it's the one most people are anxious about. There is a common misconception that you need meat for protein. The food industry has spent billions pushing that narrative, and it needs to be challenged. It's the first question every vegan must face: Where do you get your protein? We are a society obsessed with protein, but our obsession focuses on animal protein while ignoring or bypassing healthier (and often cheaper) plant proteins.

Protein is essential, and there is no denying that we need it; it is the building block of our cellular structures. Your body needs it to maintain and repair healthy tissues, bones, cartilage, and muscles. Proteins are made up of amino acids which the body uses to make enzymes (such as digestive enzymes that help you break down and absorb your food), hormones (such as epinephrine, which is important for muscle function and blood vessels; thyroxine, which is essential for thyroid function; and melatonin, which regulates your circadian rhythm).[3]

There are 21 amino acids the body needs for optimum health, nine of which are called essential because the body cannot make them, so they must be obtained from food. These essential amino acids are isoleucine, leucine, lysine, tryptophan, valine, threonine, histidine, phenylalanine and methionine. You'll find a list of these amino acids alongside food sources in the Appendix.

The reason we assume that animal products are the pinnacle of protein foods is that meat is classed as a "complete" protein because it contains all nine essential amino acids. However, it falls short in other areas: meat contains few vitamins, and no fiber or antioxidants.

But the good news is that you have options. Many plant foods contain these essential amino acids. And some contain all 21 essential amino acids. They are soybeans (edamame beans, tofu, tempeh), buckwheat, quinoa, hemp seeds and mycoprotein (mushroom protein, such as Quorn).

Shifting the protein in your diet from animal meat to plant-based proteins is one of the most powerful measures someone can take to reduce the impact on our climate.
LEONARDO DICAPRIO

You can also combine certain plant food groups to obtain all nine essential amino acids:

- Combine grains and beans or legumes: for example peanut butter and oat crackers (peanuts are legumes, not nuts), rice and lentils, pasta and kidney beans, millet and black beans, couscous and chickpeas.
- Combine nuts or seeds with legumes or beans: for example pumpkin seeds and split peas, chickpeas and tahini (also known as hummus), sunflower seeds and black-eyed beans, almonds and lentils.

You can use the above to make quick, protein-rich side dishes or salads. For example, mixing canned lentils with toasted almonds, adding a drizzle of olive oil, squeeze of lemon and a pinch of salt. You can serve this alongside a grain (rice/pasta) and some veggies (roasted, stir-fried, or raw) and ta-dah! You've got a balanced, tasty and filling meal.

HOW MUCH PROTEIN DO YOU ACTUALLY NEED?

According to experts, sedentary adults need around 0.8 g of protein for every kilo of weight, or 0.43 g of protein per pound of weight, every day.[4] This equates to around 62 g of protein per day for an adult weighing 77 kilos / 170 pounds.

How does this translate in terms of food? Here are a few examples:

- 1 cup soybeans = 28.6 g protein[5]
- 1 Beyond Burger plant-based patty = 20 g protein[6]
- 1 Impossible Burger plant-based patty = 19 g protein[7]
- 1 cup cooked lentils = 18 g protein[8]
- 1 cup cooked split peas = 16.3 g protein[9]
- 1 cup cooked chickpeas = 14.5 g protein[10]
- 1 cup cooked quinoa = 11.4 g protein[11]
- 1/4 cup cashew nuts = 7.3 g protein[12]
- 1/4 cup sesame seeds = 6.4 g protein[13]
- 1 cup cooked buckwheat = 5.7 g protein[14]
- 1/4 cup almonds = 4.9 g protein[15]
- 2 tbsp flax seeds = 2.5 g protein[16]

But protein is not only present in beans, pulses, nuts and seeds. Grains and vegetables also contain some protein. For example:

- 1 cup cooked millet = 6.1 g protein[17]
- 1 cup cooked brown rice = 5 g protein[18]
- 1 cup broccoli = 3.7 g protein[19]
- 1 cup onions = 2.6 g protein[20]
- 1 cup mushrooms = 2.5 g protein[21]
- 1 cup cooked kale = 2.5 g protein[22]
- 1 cup cooked squash = 1.7 g protein[23]

You will find a handy table in the Appendix showing good sources of plant protein. The important thing to remember is that if you eat three good meals a day made up of plant-based whole foods, you will not struggle to get enough protein for your body.

The idea that meat is the best source of protein is a fallacy. Plant proteins are healthier (because they also contain fiber, minerals, and vitamins), cheaper, and better for the environment. In the last two years, Covid and a frightening sequence of climate disasters have sent many of us to the plant-based aisle. This has scared the meat industry, which has responded by pumping out articles aiming to push people back to meat by comparing "natural" beef burgers with "unnatural" plant-based options. But even this hasn't worked: nutritionists have come out in defense of plant-meats, stating that both the Beyond Meat and Impossible Burger contain more protein and less saturated fats than beef burgers.[24]

Plant-based meat substitutes are one way to easily adjust your diet to transition toward veganism.

Here are a few other ideas to get started:

- Use tofu or tempeh instead of chicken, pork, or beef in your stir-fries. Tofu is a blank canvas when it comes to flavor - you can marinate it with herbs or spices, and then fry, roast or bake it. Then serve alongside noodles, pasta, salads...
- Replace meat with lentils, beans, or plant-based mince in your chillies and curries.
- Add chickpeas or other beans to your salads for a protein kick.
- Try jackfruit, which has a texture similar to pulled pork or shredded chicken. Jackfruit can be marinated in whatever seasonings and sauces you enjoy. Jackfruit is a great meat substitute in curries - check out my *REBEL VEGAN* recipes!
- Add hummus (or nut-based vegan cheese) to your sandwiches instead of deli meats or dairy cheese.
- Make scrambled tofu instead of scrambled eggs for breakfast.
- Try a chickpea omelette (made with gram flour) instead of an egg-based omelette.
- Try mashing chickpeas with vegan mayo or avocado for a mock tuna-mayo mix you can add to jacket potatoes or wraps.
- Fill your pittas with falafels (made from chickpeas) instead of meat or cheese.
- Try black beans instead of beef in your burritos.
- A marinated and baked portobello mushroom with avocado and vegan cheese is a delicious plant-based alternative to a beef burger.
- Have fun taste-testing the incredible variety of plant-based burgers to find one you love!

THE CONFUSION OVER CARBOHYDRATES

Carbohydrates are your body's main source of fuel. Your digestive enzymes break carbs down into glucose, which your cells convert into energy to carry out all their various functions–from moving your muscles to powering your thoughts (did you know your brain uses around 120 grams of glucose every day?[25]).

For the last decade or more, it has been increasingly fashionable to stay away from carbohydrates. This is a mistake. Not all carbohydrates are created equal–the trick is to choose the right ones. The three main types of carbohydrates are sugars, starches, and fiber. These can be split into two categories:

SIMPLE CARBOHYDRATES: The ones to limit

You'll find simple carbohydrates in fruit and cow's milk, as well as processed foods like fizzy drinks, cakes, sweets, ready meals, etc.

- Refined foods: such as white flour, white pasta, white bread, which are made from grains that have had their nutrients (such as the germ) removed.
- Added sugars: such as cane sugar, high-fructose corn syrup, glucose syrup.
- Naturally occurring sugars: fructose (found in fruits) and lactose (found in milk).
-

COMPLEX CARBOHYDRATES: The ones to indulge/good kind

You'll find complex carbohydrates in whole foods.

- Fiber–found in vegetables, whole grains, beans, legumes, fruits, nuts, and seeds.
- Starch–found in whole grains, root vegetables, beans, and pulses.

Simple carbohydrates are made up of one or two sugar molecules (mono-saccharides or di-saccharides), which are quickly absorbed by the body. Because of this, they tend to spike your blood sugar levels, disrupt insulin signalling, mess with your appetite, and increase the risk of disease.

In fact, scientists blame refined sugars for the current obesity, diabetes, and cardiovascular disease epidemics.[26] One reason for this is that diets high in refined carbohydrates cause an increase in c-reactive protein (CPR), a marker of chronic inflammation.[27]

On the other hand, complex carbohydrates are made up of three or more sugar molecules (oligo-saccharides or poly-saccharides), which are bonded together in a more complex chemical structure, and therefore broken down by the body more slowly. This means blood sugar levels remain stable, and the pancreas doesn't have to pump out a load of insulin.

Furthermore, complex carbohydrates contain vitamins and minerals that help the body stay healthy. Studies show that diets high in complex carbohydrates offer protection against many chronic diseases, including the ability to reverse existing diabetes and heart disease.[28]

Head to the Appendix to find a handy table with sources of complex carbohydrates.

FANTASTIC FIBER

The reason complex carbohydrates are better for you is that they contain plenty of healthy fiber. The fiber in whole foods helps with weight management, digestion, heart health, and even cancer prevention. Meat, fish, and dairy contain no fiber whatsoever. It is only found in plants. There are two types of fiber, both of which are beneficial: soluble and insoluble.

Soluble fiber soaks up water and turns into a gel (think about what happens when you mix water and oatmeal or chia seeds). It helps lower cholesterol because it prevents some dietary cholesterol from being absorbed. Over time, this can lower cholesterol levels. Soluble fiber also helps keep blood sugar levels stable, because it slows down the digestion of carbohydrates. What's more, it feeds the good bacteria in your gut, helping keep your digestive system healthy and your immune system strong.[29]

Insoluble fiber does not soak up water (think about what happens if you mix chopped kale with water). It acts like a broom, cleaning your digestive tract and ensuring things keep moving regularly. It adds bulk to your stools, which prevents constipation.

Although there is no fiber in meat or milk, you will find both soluble and insoluble fiber in varying proportions in all plant foods.[30]

People who eat a standard Western diet get on average 10 to 15 grams of fiber a day. This is far from the 40 grams recommended for health.[31] When you eat a plant-based diet, getting enough fiber is seldom a problem.

Carbohydrates are not the enemy, far from it! Studies show that people who eat a diet that contains plenty of complex carbohydrates from whole, natural foods (whole grains, beans, fruits and vegetables) are at a lower risk of obesity, type 2 diabetes and heart disease.[32]

Head to the Appendix for a full list of complex carbohydrates you can include in your diet.

Here are a few ways to start adding more complex carbohydrates and fiber to your day:

- Start your day with whole grains: for example, a bowl of steel-cut porridge oats (avoid instant porridge because this tends to be made from refined oats which have less fiber), granola or muesli made with whole grains, nuts and seeds (check the label and make sure that whole grains are the first ingredient and that there is little or no added sugar).
- Swap your bread for a whole grain variety: this is an effortless way to add more fiber into your day. Plus, whole grain loaves of bread are more satisfying and will keep you fuller than white bread.
- Swap your usual pasta or noodles for whole grain varieties: buckwheat noodles, whole grain spelt pasta, or even pasta made of beans or lentils, are an easy way to add more complex carbs into your life.
- Search beyond the bread aisle: Satisfy your carb craving with starchy vegetables like sweet potatoes, carrots and parsnips. They can be roasted and used in sandwiches, wraps or salads.
- Experiment with different grains: Branch out and try new things, such as quinoa, buckwheat, couscous, black rice, millet, barley. There are now tons of new and exciting bean kinds of pasta, and even couscous made from peas!

ARE FRUITS SIMPLE CARBOHYDRATES OR COMPLEX CARBOHYDRATES?

Both! Fruits contain simple carbohydrates (fructose), but they also contain fiber (especially in their skin and seeds) and other nutrients, such as antioxidants and fiber. So you can consider fruit a complex carbohydrate food, and an excellent addition to a balanced diet.

The best fruits are those that are colorful, low in sugar, and have edible peel and/or seeds (make sure you buy organic if you are not going to peel your produce), such as berries, apples, kiwis, watermelon, and papaya.

For optimum health and absorption of all the goodness in fruit, avoid juiced or fruit smoothies and eat the fruit whole. The basic rule is always to choose whole-foods over processed.

HEALTHY FATS

Before carbs were vilified, fats were held responsible for all our ills. The 80s brought us fat-free diets, but this did little to curb our globally expanding waistlines or reduce the number of heart attacks. This demonstrates that simply targeting one food group is not the answer.

Fat is not the enemy. Far from it. In fact, we need fat to function. The brain is made up mostly of fat. The protective layer around some neurons, known as the myelin sheath, is made up of fat. Cell membranes are made up of fat. Our liver needs fat in order to produce hormones.

But of course, just like carbohydrates and proteins, the quality of fat is important. Certain fats are best avoided, while others should take pride of place on your plate.

There are four main types of fat: saturated fats, trans-saturated fats, monounsaturated fats and polyunsaturated fats. The first two are usually solid at room temperature (like animal fat, butter or coconut oil), while the second two are usually liquid (like vegetable oil).

The accepted and over-simplified position is that saturated fats are bad because they increase cholesterol, while unsaturated fats are good because they can lower cholesterol. Both these statements are not as black and white as they seem.

When it comes to saturated fat and cholesterol, only 20% of the cholesterol in the body comes from food, the rest is produced by the body.[33] However, eating too much saturated fat causes a hike in LDL cholesterol (that's the "bad" cholesterol that increases the risk of heart disease and strokes). The standard Western diet contains a lot of saturated fat because of its high proportion of meat, dairy and eggs. That being said, not all saturated fats are bad–some are actually good for you. Coconut oil, for example, contains saturated fat alongside lauric acid, which increases HDL cholesterol (this is the good type of cholesterol that lowers the risk of heart disease).[34]

Looking at unsaturated fats, their health halo is not quite as bright as we might have been led to believe. Most of the unsaturated fats we consume come from vegetable oils like canola, corn, and soybean. These crops are either heavily sprayed with pesticides or genetically modified (in the US, 94% of soybean crops, 95% of canola crops, and 92% of corn crops are GMO[35]). As a result, the oils contain residues of pesticides and fertilizers, which have been shown to damage gut health[36] and are implicated in cancer (in 2015, the International Agency for Research on Cancer classified glyphosate, the most widely used herbicide in the world, as a Group 2A carcinogen[37]).

The way these oils are made doesn't bode well for their nutrient content either. Unlike olive oil or coconut oil, which can be obtained simply by pressing the fruit, vegetable oils have to undergo a lot of chemical processing (they have to be heated, mixed with solvents to extract the oils, then deodorized and treated to improve the smell, color, and flavor[38]). As we have shown, the more processing food has to go through, the less beneficial it is to health.

There's more. These oils are high in Omega-6. Which on the surface sounds good. We've all heard about the benefits of Omega-3 and Omega-6 fatty acids. We need both because the body does not produce either. Both are brain-healthy nutrients and are needed to help the body fight inflammation. But only in the right proportions.

The ideal ratio of Omega-3 to Omega-6 is between 1:1 and 1:3. In other words, we need to consume more or less the same amount of each, or just a little more Omega-6 than Omega-3. The standard Western diet, with its take-out foods and fried foods, is too rich in Omega-6. We're eating around twenty times more Omega-6 than Omega-3. The result is higher levels of chronic inflammation.

Your body uses Omega-6 and Omega-3 to make molecules called eicosanoids that are involved in the body's inflammation responses. The eicosanoids made from Omega-6 are pro-inflammatory, while those made from Omega-3 are anti-inflammatory. Both are needed because as we saw earlier, inflammation (when acute) is a beneficial action. But too much Omega-6 means more pro-inflammatory molecules are created in the body, and this can lead to chronic inflammation, which increases the risk of diseases such as cardiovascular disease, obesity, and Alzheimer's disease.[39]

To counter this, we need to reduce our intake of Omega-6 and eat more foods high in Omega-3. We'll take a closer look at Omega-3 in the Micronutrients section. In the Appendix section, you'll find a list of healthy fats to include in your diet.

Ways to add healthy fats to your diet:
- Swap your vegetable oils for cold-pressed olive oil, coconut oil, walnut oil, avocado oil, sesame oil, or flaxseed oil. Use coconut oil or avocado oil for cooking (both have a high smoke point, which makes them safe to heat at higher temperatures, and the others for making dressings or adding flavor to your dishes.
- Eat more avocados! Have it on toast, add to your salads, or blend with cacao powder and maple syrup to make a quick chocolate mousse.
- Snack on nuts and seeds.
- Roast nuts or seeds with spices or herbs, and add them to your meals for extra texture, flavor, and healthy fats.

CHOLESTEROL: GOOD OR BAD?

Cholesterol is a substance mired in misinformation. It isn't as simple as "cholesterol is bad." The truth is that the liver produces cholesterol to help build healthy cell membranes and hormones. But when too much cholesterol is obtained from our diet, problems arise.

There are two types of cholesterol: LDL (low-density lipoprotein) and HDL (high-density lipoprotein).

LDL cholesterol is known as "bad cholesterol" because it contributes to atherosclerosis (clogged arteries). HDL cholesterol is known as "good cholesterol" because it helps clear LDL cholesterol from blood vessels.

When cholesterol levels are measured, doctors will first look at total cholesterol, and then look at the ratio of LDL to HDL cholesterol to get a more accurate view of a person's health. A higher proportion of HDL cholesterol indicates a lower risk of heart disease. Ideally, total blood cholesterol should be less than 150 mg/dL (milligrams per deciliter) and the ratio of total cholesterol to HDL should be less than 4 to 1. However, the average American's ratio is 5 to 1, and almost 107 million Americans have cholesterol levels greater than 200 mg/dL. The average cholesterol level of coronary heart disease victims is 225 mg/dL.

The biggest source of cholesterol in our diet is animal products. Meat, dairy and eggs raise cholesterol levels and increase the risk of cardiovascular disease. On the other hand, whole plant-based foods do the opposite: their fiber slows the absorption of dietary cholesterol and reduces the amount of cholesterol produced by the liver, leading to a reduced risk of cardiovascular disease.[40]

ANOTHER PIECE OF THE PUZZLE: GUT HEALTH

No journey towards health is complete without addressing your digestive system and the bacteria that reside there.

Your gut is a foundational part of your health. We've talked about how your immune system can become disrupted and trigger chronic inflammation in response to certain foods. One of the best ways to improve health is to bring your immune system back into balance. And a key part of that is looking after your digestive system.

We see ourselves as complete and fully-formed humans, but that isn't the whole story. The body is made up of trillions of bacterial microorganisms. In fact, these cells outnumber human cells by 10 to 1.[41] While this might sound a bit crude, these bacteria should be celebrated because they work around the clock to keep you healthy. They are your first line of defense against disease.

Your immune system comes to life the moment you are born. When you passed through the birth canal, you became seeded with bacteria from your mother. This bacteria, along with the bacteria in breast milk and the germs you naturally came into contact with in your early childhood, made up your unique bacterial fingerprint. From birth, these microbes taught your immune system how to respond to viruses, germs, and other threats. How well you can defend yourself against illness depends very much on having a strong population of bacteria.

The largest and most important concentration of bacteria is found in your gut. This is your immune system's piece de resistance – in fact, some scientists believe 80% of the immune system is located there. Gut microbes break down food into usable molecules, process indigestible carbohydrates (fiber) to produce essential vitamins, and trigger the appropriate immune-protective responses.

This means that if your gut is compromised, so is your immune system. The good news is that we know what damages the gut, and how to strengthen it.

Your gut lining is the barrier between your body and undigested food. When it is healthy, only food processed into useful molecules can pass through. If the gut lining becomes weak (a condition known as leaky gut or increased gut permeability), it can allow undigested particles to leak into your bloodstream. When this happens, your immune system recognizes these particles as foreign and launches an attack. The result is increased inflammation and changes in the gut's normal bacterial balance, which can lead to digestive problems and chronic disease.

Most people have leaky gut or bacterial imbalance to some degree, and our modern lifestyles are to blame. Here's how:

- Diet and inflammatory foods: The standard Western diet is high in sugar, fats, and processed foods that disrupt the gut's bacterial balance. Studies show that high meat diets cause gut dysbiosis[42] (a term that describes when bad bacteria outnumber the good bacteria).
- Pesticide residues: The chemicals used to grow our food has a negative impact on our gut. Research shows that even at allowed "safe" levels, glyphosate reduces good bacteria (particularly lactobacillus bacteria, which help fight inflammation), while increasing bad bacteria (such as prevotella bacteria, which is associated with overactive immune responses and low-grade inflammation).[43]
- Antibiotics: They're useful, but they destroy all bacteria, including the good ones.
- Ultra-sanitized environments: Our love of disinfecting everything means we are less exposed to naturally occurring bacteria.

- Lack of fiber: Fiber feeds the good bacteria in your gut. What's more, not eating enough fiber leads to constipation - and when waste lingers in the gut, this causes gut bacteria imbalances that weaken the intestinal lining.

DO YOU HAVE A LEAKY GUT?

Here are signs you could do with giving your gut a helping hand:

- Skin conditions such as acne, psoriasis, eczema
- Acid reflux
- Allergies
- Frequent illness
- Mood issues such as brain fog, anxiety, depression
- Fatigue
- Excess weight
- Swollen, red, or painful joints
- Digestive discomfort such as bloating, diarrhea, or constipation
- Trouble sleeping

It is possible to rebalance your gut.

It takes a simple, two-step process:

1. Avoid inflammatory foods: This means reducing your consumption of processed foods and avoiding meat and dairy. The good news is you've picked up this book at exactly the right time!
2. Include gut-friendly foods: This means foods that contain beneficial bacteria (fermented or probiotic foods) and foods that contain gut-friendly fiber (plant-based whole foods).

You will find a handy list of gut-friendly fermented foods, and tips to add them to your diet, in the Appendix.

Now that we know about the macronutrients you need to add to your diet to maintain your best health, let's take a look at which micronutrients will put a spring in your step.

MICRONUTRIENTS

These little powerhouses are essential for good health. Your body uses vitamins, minerals, and antioxidants to support many of its functions.

The first thing I will say about micronutrients is this: if you eat a diet made up of mostly plant foods, you will get the micronutrients you need for optimum health. That being said, when you switch to veganism, it is important to focus on certain key nutrients to ensure you get adequate amounts.

In this section, I'll tackle the main ones. In the appendix, you will find a table showing all the essential vitamins and minerals and where you can find them.

OMEGA-3

Omega-3 fatty acids are essential for maintaining and protecting cell membranes, particularly the brain, eyes, and cardiovascular system, as well as supporting your endocrine system (the network of glands that produce your hormones).[44] Your body uses Omega-3 to make molecules that help your immune system fight inflammation, making it a very useful tool to lower chronic inflammation and get your body back into balance.

Most people hear "Omega-3" and instantly think "fish oil." But did you know that fish get their Omega-3 from plants in the form of algae? The problem with prioritizing fish and fish oils to obtain enough Omega-3 is that these products also contain chemicals (heavy metals and pollutants like dioxin, mercury, and microplastics) that, ironically, put your health in danger. That's not to mention the environmental, ethical, and animal cruelty issues surrounding fish farming.

There are three Omega-3 fatty acids:

- Alpha-linolenic acid (ALA): found in plants such as flaxseed, which the body converts into EPA and DHA.
- Eicosapentaenoic acid (EPA): found in fish and fish oils
- Docosahexaenoic (DHA): found in fish and fish oils

Fish obtain their ALA Omega-3 from algae and then convert it to EPA and DHA. This conversion can be difficult for the human body, which is why some people insist that fish is essential to obtain enough Omega-3. Let me show you why this is not entirely true.

According to research from Cochrane University, EPA and DHA from oily fish and fish oil supplements have little or no effect on heart health.[45] On the other hand, a review of studies published in the British Journal of Nutrition found that ALA from plant foods helps reduce the risk of heart disease.[46] Put it another way: plant-based Omega-3 is better for you.

You can obtain your Omega-3 straight from the source (plants) instead of the middle man (fish). In fact, one study found that people on vegan diets obtain, on average, more than the recommended intake of Omega-3.[47]

Here are seven foods that are high in Omega-3:

- Chia seeds: 4,915 mg of Omega-3 per ounce (28 g)
- Hemp seeds: 6000 mg Omega-3 per ounce (28 g)
- Flax seeds: 6,388 mg of Omega-3 per ounce (28 g)
- Walnuts: 2,542 mg of Omega-3 per ounce (28 g)
- Algae oil supplement: Typically 300-500 mg of Omega-3 per capsule
- Perilla oil (made from perilla seeds, often used in Korean cuisine): 9,000 mg of Omega-3 per tablespoon (14 g)

Other plant foods also contain Omega-3, for example:

- Kidney beans: 300 mg per cup
- Brussels sprouts: 270 mg per cup
- Squash: 190 mg per cup
- Collard greens: 180 mg per cup
- Cauliflower: 210 mg per cup
- Chickpeas: 70 mg per cup
- Pumpkin seeds: 160 mg per cup
- Sunflower seeds: 120 mg per cup

Ways to add these to your diet:

- Make a chia pudding and have it for breakfast or a filling snack.
- Sprinkle chia seeds, hemp seeds, or flax seeds onto your breakfast cereal or other meals.
- Add chia seeds, hemp seeds, or flax seeds to your smoothies.
- Make energy balls or granola bars using chia seeds, hemp seeds, flax seeds, and/or walnuts.
- Toast walnuts and add to salads or have a handful as a snack.
- Use perilla oil instead of other oils (this would work well in a stir-fry or curry).
- Roast cauliflower or squash with curry spices and serve as a side dish, or blend them into a creamy soup.
- Sauté collard greens with a little garlic for a healthy side dish, or add to stir-fries.

B12

B12 is essential for the body's nervous system, red blood cells, and making DNA. Not getting enough can lead to megaloblastic anemia, where the bone marrow produces abnormal and immature red blood cells. If this happens, blood cells cannot deliver enough oxygen through the body. This leads to fatigue, lightheadedness, and irregular heartbeat. Left untreated, it can lead to irreparable nerve damage.[48]

This is the one nutrient vegans need to worry about because in today's world B12 is found exclusively in animal protein. This means you will need to get your B12 through supplementation. A B12 supplement is absolutely non-negotiable as you transition to a vegan diet. Check out the box below for the story of B12.

Thankfully, many vegan foods, such as soy products, plant-based milks, and cereals, are fortified with B12. The recommended intake of B12 is 2.4 micrograms a day, so check the label to see how much these foods provide. The simplest, most economical and convenient option is to take a good quality supplement.

Vegan sources of B12 include:

- Yeast extract (such as Marmite)
- Nutritional yeast (great for adding a cheesy flavor without dairy!)
- Breakfast cereals fortified with B12
- Plant milks fortified with B12
- Soy products fortified with B12
- ESSENTIAL: Good quality vegan multivitamin containing B12

Aim for a daily intake of 3 micrograms of B12 from food, or supplement at least 10 micrograms of B12 every day. While this is higher than the recommended intake, it will ensure you get enough of this nutrient. Your body only absorbs around 10 micrograms from a 500 microgram B12 supplement.[49]

For this reason, PETA recommends either eating enough fortified foods to obtain 3 micrograms per day or taking a daily cyanocobalamin B12 supplement (which your body converts to the two active forms of B12, methylcobalamin and adenosylcobalamin).[50]

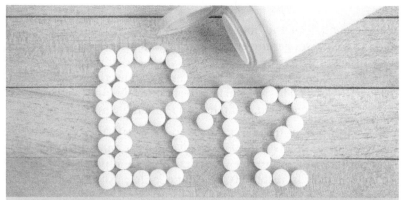

THE MISSING LINK: THE MYSTERY OF NATURE'S MISSING VITAMIN

The elusive and mysterious B12 is the only nutrient vegans cannot obtain from a fully plant-based diet. It's the missing link and it has always both bothered and intrigued me. It made me wonder how our mostly plant-based ancestors survived and evolved. And I felt a little cheated by Mother Nature!

So I did a bit of digging and found interesting explanations, as well as a theory accepted by most historians for our ecosystem's glaring omission.

B12 is not made by plants or animals, but by bacteria that blanket the earth. Basically, it is in the dirt (or soil). Before modern hygiene practices, traces of this bacteria from water, soil, and vegetables would get onto our fingers and into our mouths and guts, giving us the B12 we needed to survive and evolve - regardless of whether our ancestors had the methods or skills to kill wild animals (which they often didn't).

Our closest relatives, gorillas, get their B12 from accidentally eating soil (which contains bacteria) as part of their plant-based diet. Early humans got plenty of B12 from soil and from drinking water from rivers and streams that contain B12 and B12 producing bacteria. However, in today's sanitized world, water is commonly chlorinated to eliminate bacteria. This is positive, as we don't get cholera from our water supplies. But the downside is we don't get B12 either. What's more, due to intensive agricultural processes and over-farming, our soils no longer contain B12 producing bacteria. This is a problem for us and for animals.

Cattle naturally get B12 from clumps of dirt around grassroots; chickens get their B12 from pecking soil for worms and insects. But farmed animals do not graze. They are kept indoors and never see the soil in their lifetime, so they would be deficient in B12 if it wasn't for supplementation. These artificial conditions make the "vegan is unnatural" argument seem somewhat ironic.

Did you know that 90% of B12 supplements are given to farmed animals? They are supplementing too.

In other words, people who eat meat simply receive B12 from the supplements given to the animals. Isn't it far better to simply take a B12 supplement and cut out the middle-man—or cow?

By the way, it's not just vegans who are at risk of B12 deficiency. The Framingham Offspring Study found that 39% of the population has either low or very low B12 levels. Interestingly, there was no difference between those who ate meat and poultry and those who didn't. The people with the highest levels of B12 were those who ate B12 fortified foods and those who took a B12 supplement.

CALCIUM

"The human body has no more need for cows' milk than it does for dogs' milk, horses' milk, or giraffes' milk."

DR. MICHAEL KLAPER[51]

Calcium is vital for strong bones and much more besides. Your heart, muscles and nerves also require calcium in order to function properly. Calcium alongside Vitamin D (which your body needs to absorb calcium and make use of it) might even have a protective effect against cancer, heart disease, and high blood pressure.[52]

We have been repeatedly told that the only way we can build strong bones is by consuming dairy. It is time to shatter this myth. The reason milk contains calcium is that green plants pull calcium out of the soil through their roots and into their leaves.

Here again, cows are the middle-man; they eat the grass, we drink their milk. We have another option–we can go straight to the source. I don't mean to suggest you start eating grass, but leafy greens are a tasty alternative!

You need around 1,000 milligrams of calcium a day. Many vegan foods, such as plant-based milk, are fortified with calcium–many even contain more calcium than milk!

You can get all the calcium you need from leafy greens (like Swiss chard, broccoli, and kale), as well as other plant foods (listed below). This offers a double benefit: the calcium without the animal cruelty, and with added fiber and antioxidants that support health (whereas a cup of milk contains saturated fat that increases your risk of chronic disease[53]).

Plant-based sources of calcium include:[54]
- Tofu: 774 mg of calcium per 4 ounces (110 g)
- Collard greens: 267 mg of calcium per cup
- Swiss chard: 101 mg of calcium per cup
- Sesame seeds: 1404 mg of calcium per cup
- Kale: 93 mg of calcium per cup
- Bok choi: 158 mg of calcium per cup
- Almonds: 240 mg of calcium per cup
- Cabbage: 63 mg of calcium per cup
- Figs: 17 mg of calcium per medium fig
- Lentils: 37 mg of calcium per cup
- Bread and plant-based milk with added calcium (check the label for calcium amount)

Tips to add more calcium to your diet:

- Eat your greens: Include a portion of greens such as kale or collard greens in your day by adding them to stir-fries, sautéing them in olive oil and garlic, or steaming and adding to pasta for a filling green meal.
- Eat tofu: You can marinate it in maple syrup, ginger, and turmeric, or different spices, then fry, bake or roast and serve alongside vegetables and grains. Alternatively, add to your curries and stews, or try scrambled tofu instead of eggs. You can also add silken tofu to creamy soups and smoothies for an extra protein kick that will also deliver the calcium you need.
- Snack on dried figs and almonds.
- Make hummus by blending chickpeas, tahini (sesame seed paste), olive oil and garlic. Keep this in your fridge as a handy snack or tasty sandwich spread.
- Choose plant-based milk with added calcium (but check the label and avoid varieties with added sugar and preservatives).

IRON

Another nutrient we are told we need animal products for, and another nutrient we can get more efficiently from plants. Iron is essential for maintaining healthy blood by helping the body to produce red blood cells. If you don't get enough iron, the result is iron deficiency anemia. This condition affects between 4 and 5 million Americans every year and is the most common nutritional deficiency in the world.[55]

All animals get their iron from...you know the answer already: plants! Therefore, we can get iron from both plants and animals. But balance is key. Too much heme iron can trigger the production of free radicals, which damage cells, trigger disease, cause premature ageing, and has been linked to several types of cancer.[56] To understand this better, let's look at the two forms of iron: heme and non-heme.

Heme iron is found only in animal products (meat, poultry and seafood). Non-heme iron is found in plant foods (whole grains, nuts, seeds, leafy greens, and legumes). The body absorbs heme iron from animal products regardless of its current level of iron. This means your body absorbs it from animal products, whether you need iron or not. Heme iron bypasses your body's attempts to control iron absorption. This can lead to high iron levels (and the formation of free radicals that I mentioned above, leading to a higher risk of premature ageing and some cancers).

On the other hand, your body can adjust its absorption of non-heme iron depending on your iron levels–it is more absorbable when you need it, and less absorbable if your levels are too high. This means you can eat iron-rich plants without worrying about iron toxicity. And this is what gives non-heme iron a definite advantage over heme iron. Another win for plants. Now I know why my mother always said to finish my greens!

When it comes to iron supplementation, it is best avoided unless under the instruction of your doctor. You can get plenty of iron from a balanced plant-based diet. The recommended amount of iron is 8 milligrams per day for adult men and 18 milligrams per day for adult women.[57]

The richest sources of iron include:[58]

- Soybeans: 8.8 mg of iron per cup
- Lentils: 6.5 mg of iron per cup
- Spinach: 6.4 mg of iron per cup
- Sesame seeds: 21.6 mg of iron per cup
- Chickpeas: 4.7 mg of iron per cup
- Olives: 4.4 mg of iron per cup
- Kidney beans: 3.9 mg of iron per cup
- Swiss chard: 3.9 mg of iron per cup
- Black beans: 3.6 mg of iron per cup
- Pumpkin seeds: 2.8 mg of iron per cup
- Green peas: 2.8 mg of iron per cup
- Cumin: 2.7 mg of iron per 2 teaspoons
- Beet greens: 2.7 mg of iron per cup
- Asparagus: 1.6 mg of iron per cup
- Leeks: 1.1 mg of iron per cup

Ideas to include more iron into your diet:

- Use soybeans in your chillies, salads and stews.
- Toast pumpkin seeds and make a healthy trail mix (with roasted nuts and dried fruit) you can snack on.
- Make a cumin-flavored dish, for example by sprinkling cumin onto squash or sweet potatoes and roasting, or adding to hummus or bean dips for a spicy twist.
- Snack on olives or make an olive tapenade to snack on and add to your sandwiches.
- Add lentils to your lunchtime salad for extra protein and iron.
- Make a tahini (sesame paste) dressing and drizzle it on your salads or use it as a vegetable dip.

ZINC

Zinc is another essential nutrient for your health. It plays an important role in many processes, for example keeping your immune system strong (which is why you'll often find it in many over the counter cold remedies[59]), helping wound healing, and even sharpening your senses of taste and smell (very important for tasting and smelling the delicious plant-based food you'll be making as part of your journey towards veganism!). Zinc is also vital for a healthy pregnancy and helps growth and development during infancy.

This is another nutrient that we traditionally think of as only available from meat and dairy. However, a well-planned vegan diet provides adequate amounts of zinc. Researchers at the Medical Journal of Australia found that people on a plant-based diet can absorb and retain zinc better. What's more, their research indicates vegans are at no greater risk of zinc deficiency than non-vegans.[60]

The recommended daily intake of zinc is 11 milligrams per day for adult men and 8 milligrams a day for adult women.[61]

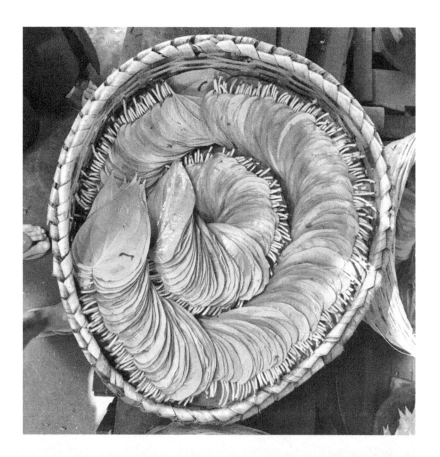

Plant-based sources of zinc include:[62]

- Spinach: 1.4 mg of zinc per cup
- Asparagus: 1.1 mg of zinc per cup
- Shiitake mushrooms: 2 mg of zinc per cup
- Sesame seeds: 11.2 mg of zinc per cup
- Quinoa: 2.7 mg of zinc per cup
- Pumpkin seeds: 10 mg of zinc per cup
- Chickpeas: 2.5 mg of zinc per cup
- Lentils: 2.5 mg of zinc per cup
- Cashew nuts: 9.2 mg of zinc per cup
- Tofu: 1.8 mg of zinc per 4 ounces (110g)
- Green peas: 1.6 mg of zinc per cup
- Oats: 6 mg of zinc per cup
- Squash: 0.7 mg of zinc per cup
- Broccoli: 0.7 mg of zinc per cup
- Swiss chard: 0.6 mg of zinc per cup
- Miso paste: 0.5 mg of zinc per tablespoon

Ideas to add more zinc to your life:

- Use shiitake mushrooms instead of chestnut mushrooms in your stir-fries and curries.
- Pan fry shiitake mushrooms with tamari sauce, soy sauce, or rosemary, and pile on top of sourdough bread for an epic zinc-boosting brunch dish.
- Prepare some homemade hummus using chickpeas and tahini - keep it in your fridge for a handy snack or just to dollop onto your salads and into sandwiches.
- Snack on roasted cashew nuts or pumpkin seeds.
- Try quinoa instead of brown rice or pasta.
- Start your day with a bowl of porridge, or add a handful of oats to your smoothies.
- Make a quick Asian-style dressing by mixing miso paste, a little water and a squeeze of lemon to liven up your veggies or use it to marinate tofu.

VITAMIN D

Also known as the sunshine vitamin, vitamin D is essential for many of the body's processes. For one, it is essential for strong bones because it helps your body absorb and use calcium. It also has a role in blood sugar control.

Some studies have found that vitamin D deficiency can increase the risk of developing diabetes, because it leads to impaired insulin control.[63] But perhaps even more important, vitamin D is essential for the body to produce mature and well-functioning white blood cells (these are your first line of defense against infection). A review of studies by the British Medical Journal found that vitamin D supplementation can protect against acute respiratory tract infections[64]--something that is particularly relevant right now to help fight Covid.

Very few foods naturally contain vitamin D, and most of them are animal foods, such as salmon, sardines, tuna, cow's milk and eggs. But even these foods do not deliver adequate amounts to save us from vitamin D deficiency.

In the US, where meat and dairy are consumed in large amounts, 41.6% of the population has vitamin D deficiency.[65] Humans naturally produce vitamin D when skin cells are exposed to sunlight. But with many of us staying indoors and wearing sunscreen, we rarely get enough sunlight to top up our levels.

So what's the answer?

Eating foods that are enriched with vitamin D, and taking a good-quality supplement. Make sure you choose a vegan brand because conventional vitamin D supplements are derived from lanolin (a fatty substance found in lamb's wool).

To avoid deficiency, the National Institutes of Health recommend an intake of 12 micrograms (or 600 IU - international units) per day for adults.[66]

SOURCES OF VITAMIN D:[67]
- White mushrooms (exposed to UV light to boost vitamin D concentration): 18.4 mg of vitamin D per cup
- Soy, almond, and oat milk fortified with vitamin D: 2.5 to 3.6 mg of vitamin D per cup
- Cereal fortified with vitamin D: 2 mg of vitamin D per serving (check the label)
- ESSENTIAL: Good quality vegan vitamin D supplement (check the label)

BEGIN PUTTING IT INTO PRACTICE

Becoming a *REBEL VEGAN* involves challenging the dominant belief system and seeing through the profit-driven farming industry's claims about meat and dairy being healthy. I hope I've been able to convey to you in this chapter just how nutritious a plant-based diet can be.

Meat and dairy are not these magical foods that offer us everything we need for health–far from it. In fact, we can get everything we need from plant foods.

You might be wondering how this looks in practice. The trick here is to avoid overcomplicating it. As long as you make sure all macronutrients are present in your meals, you'll give yourself what you need for optimum health. A good way to visualize it is to fill half your plate with vegetables, and split the other half between complex carbohydrates and plant protein, then use healthy fats to flavor your dishes (for example by throwing on a handful of toasted seeds, or making a creamy dressing using nut or seed butters).

In the next chapter you'll find my handy 4-step program to transition to veganism. You've got the nutrition knowledge, now it's the fun part: putting it into practice. Let's start veganizing!

LOSING WEIGHT ON A VEGAN DIET

Q. What do you call someone who can't stick with a diet?
A. A desserter.

This is a guilt-free space, but... I think it won't come as a surprise when I tell you that we have put on weight during the pandemic (on average half a stone or 7 pounds[68]), because of extra stress and comfort eating. Not only is this bad for our morale, it also puts us in danger of getting sick.

Weight gain is one of the big factors in our global disease epidemics. Research shows people with excess weight are at a higher risk of diabetes, heart disease, cancer,[69] and the coronavirus. Even modest weight gain can lead to an elevated risk of hospitalization from Covid.[70]

The good news is that a vegan diet can help you shed excess weight and any Covid kilos you might have gained. Here's how:

MORE FIBER:
Fiber slows down the digestion of carbohydrates and sugar, which leads to more stable blood sugar levels and better appetite control. In other words, when you eat more plant foods, you won't feel as hungry between meal times, which leads to less snacking between meals and therefore better weight management.

PLANTS HELP YOUR BODY DETOX:
Your body is very clever. When there are too many toxins for it to process, because of pollution, stress and processed food, it stores them somewhere safe where they can do less damage–your fat cells. One of your main detoxification pathways is your digestive system. Thanks to increased fiber from plants, your bowel movements become regular, and this helps your body get rid of toxins. The result is gradual, sustainable, healthy weight loss.

ANTIOXIDANTS:
Plants are Mother Nature's medicines. Brightly colored fruits, vegetables, herbs, and spices are packed with plant pigments that act as antioxidants in the body. Antioxidants help your body neutralize free radicals and toxins. This helps your body release toxins and therefore helps you shed any excess weight.

IT'S A LIFESTYLE, NOT A DIET:

Diets don't work - they are rooted in short-term strategies that deliver short term results. The only thing we want to do when we're on a diet is to stop being on a diet. This diet mindset leads to disordered eating and disconnection with your body and your appetite.

A plant-based diet, on the other hand, is rooted in choosing foods that do your body, and the planet, good.

This is a game-changer.

It gives you the opportunity to create a diet that supports your body, tastes great, and helps you lose weight without counting calories or restricting.

I ALWAYS SAY THAT VEGANISM IS NOT ABOUT RESTRICTION, BUT RATHER ABOUT BUILDING YOUR BEST LIFE.

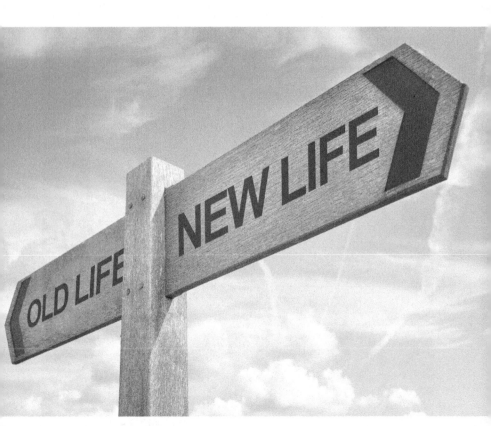

WHAT ABOUT KETO?

We've all heard about the weight-loss benefits of a meat-centric ketogenic diet. But these results are inflated as a marketing tactic. The truth is that you'll lose more weight and be healthier by switching to a plant-based diet. This has been confirmed by a study comparing weight loss from a keto diet and a vegan diet. Participants who ate a carbohydrate-rich plant-based diet ate more food but lost body fat and retained muscle, while those who followed a meat-rich ketogenic diet ate less food but retained fat while losing muscle.

The researchers attributed these results to the fact that plant foods contain more fiber. Fiber helps keep you fuller for longer, improves your gut health, and supports one of your body's main detox pathways (your digestive tract), all of which helps you to release excess weight.[71]

So you see, a vegan diet is your friend when it comes to healthy, sustainable weight loss!

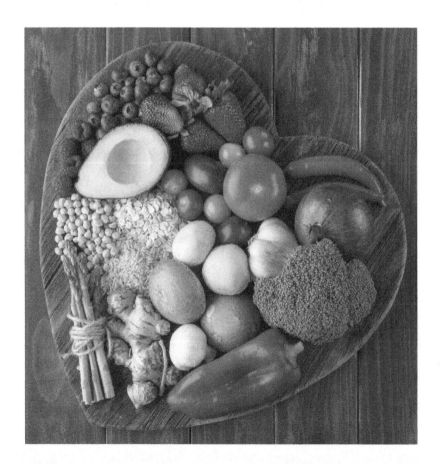

PRACTICAL WEIGHT-LOSS TIPS:

- **Fill up on fiber**. Satisfy your hunger by going for a second helping of greens or grains. The extra fiber will keep you full and help your body release excess weight.

- **Eat enough protein**. High-protein foods are the most filling foods and therefore help you manage your appetite. Add beans or tofu to your meals, snack on nuts or seeds, or add a scoop of vegan protein powder to your smoothies.

- **Start your day with a tall glass of water**. We often mistake thirst for hunger. Staying well hydrated ensures that you don't feel like snacking between meals. What's more, it helps your kidneys to flush out toxins, and this can help shift excess weight.

- **Limit processed food**. They contain a lot of sugar and fat which means we tend to over-eat them (because they taste good!) and then gain weight. Focus on whole foods instead. Go to the Appendix for a list of simple, tasty, healthy swaps to common processed foods.

- **Read the label**. Ingredients are listed in order of proportion. If sugar is the first, second, or third ingredient listed, leave that food on the shelf. If the ingredients sound like a chemistry experiment, it means the food is heavily processed and is best avoided.

- **Plan ahead**. Stock your fridge with healthy snacks you can quickly grab if a craving hits you. Hummus and vegetables, peanut butter and oat crackers, nuts and seeds, and homemade granola bars are all good options that will nourish you while helping you avoid processed foods.

- **Slow and steady wins the race.** You did not put weight on overnight, and it will take your body a little time to let go of the excess weight. Be patient and kind with yourself.

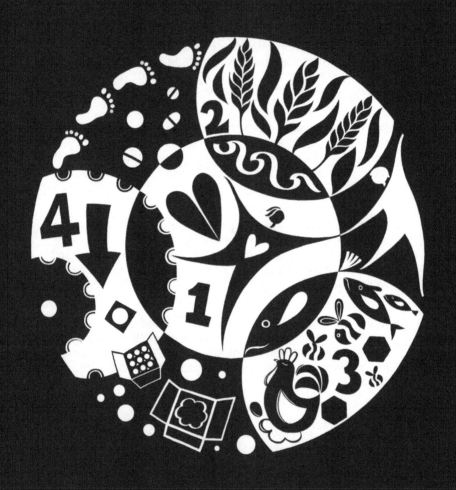

4

FOUR STEPS TO VEGAN:

REBEL VEGINNER'S GUIDE

You can't go back and change the beginning,
but you can start where you are and change the
ending.
C. S. LEWIS

Now for the fun part–putting your knowledge into practice. After all, knowledge is power, but only when it translates into action does it make a difference–as compassion without action is just observation.

The Rebel Veginner's Guide introduces an easy and engaging program on how to get animal products out of your diet and embrace a life that is in line with your values. I have organized it so each step and meal time is supported with fun and simple recipes at the back of this book.

At each stage, please check out the corresponding recipes in Chapter 9 to help keep you motivated and inspire lasting change.

I always say veganism–like life –is a journey. So grab my hand, and let's start this new adventure. There is no time like the present!

LASTING CHANGE

Q: How many meat-eaters does it take to change a light bulb?
A: None. They prefer to stay in the dark!

The best way to make changes and stick to them is to go slowly, especially when you're changing something as integral as your diet. Gradually swapping one animal product at a time gives your body and mind time to adjust to new flavors and nutrients. I've designed the *REBEL VEGAN* 4-week program to reduce your animal intake while remaining motivated, feeling supported and informed, and enjoying fabulous food.

While the steps are broken down into weeks, you have the option of going at your own pace–you're in the drivers seat. Some might race through, others might stop and pause while adjusting and finding their feet. Once you feel comfortable with each step, you can move on to the next one. In this way, you make sure you create your own journey towards the vegan you want to be.

With this unique approach, you can go as far along the vegan spectrum as you feel happy, and stop and start at any stage. You're in the driver's seat to fine-tune your diet and create your best life. If you are coming at this as a vegetarian, you only need to tackle the first step of this program to create a fully sustainable and cruelty-free life.

The goal of this guide is to be inclusive, flexible, and as guilt-free as possible. I developed this program for you to be emboldened and confident to find your own sweet spot. Although I encourage you to push yourself, only you can decide on your pace and how far you can go within your unique circumstances.

For change to last, you have to make it work for your lifestyle. There is a balance to be struck between your own driving forces, conscience, and circumstances. Of course, you have the option to go cold turkey, and while that works well for some, it doesn't sound gentle or cruelty-free!

When I first became vegan, I occasionally ate animal products at family events before my official "coming out." At home, I stopped stocking animal foods and gradually eliminated them from my kitchen cupboards and fridge. Slowly I got to know new recipes, new shops, and new restaurants. This is how I developed my unique and adaptable 4-week program. I was the first guinea pig!

Any effort you make to move further along the diet spectrum towards veganism to become more plant-based should be applauded. It will improve your health, reduce cruelty, and help create a more sustainable future.

You are becoming the change that you want to see.

BEFORE YOU BEGIN...

How many times have you started something (a diet, a health program, a course) only to give up before you've even got halfway? Don't feel bad, this happens to so many people, and all for one main reason: lack of proper planning. Yes, it's a cliché but it's true–failing to plan is planning to fail.

And by planning, I don't just mean looking at your schedule and deciding when to go food shopping. I mean taking the time to fully connect with where you are now and where you want to be, to think about the potential challenges you will face so you can decide in advance how you will deal with them, and to start designing a routine that makes your new habits second nature.

Everyone has their preference when it comes to brainstorming. I get my best ideas by either walking or cycling in nature. Maybe you prefer to sit in front of an Excel spreadsheet, or to use a large piece of paper and lots of colored pens, or just record voice notes–whatever works for you.

Here are a few questions to think about before you embark on this 4-week transition.

- **Time management:** Block some time to begin your journey. Look at your weekly schedule and workout when you have spare time and when you have spare energy. Block these times in your diary - these are the moments when you'll be able to explore new aisles in the supermarket, try new recipes. Remember this is an adventure: make it fun!
- **Your current diet:** Now that you know more about the macro and micronutrients you need, how does your current way of eating measure up? How is the standard Western diet affecting you? (excess weight, tiredness, mood swings, diabetes, troubles sleeping, digestive issues...) Ask yourself what might happen if you don't make a change?
- **Your new diet:** Using the above answers as a guide, what benefits will veganism bring to you? How will you feel physically and emotionally thanks to this new lifestyle?
- **Preparing for and overcoming obstacles:** We all have triggers–what are yours? What situations might make you turn to habitual food patterns? How can you avoid this? For example, your trigger might be a looming deadline which sends you straight to the doughnut counter; or maybe you are a people-pleaser and worry that you might fall in with your friends' food preferences. Solutions might be that you keep some healthy vegan snacks in your office, or research vegan-friendly restaurants or cafes in your area. Thinking about how you would respond to possible triggers will help you stick to your plant-based diet even when the going gets tough.
- **Keep your "why" in mind:** Remember your driving forces. What are your hopes, dreams and goals as you transition to veganism?

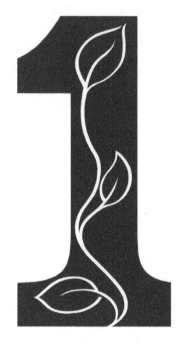

WEEK 1
START THE DAY THE RIGHT WAY!

Let's jump in! Breakfast is the most important meal of the day, so let's start here and make it vegan. If you are already vegetarian, this is your first and final step towards veganism. If you are coming to this from a standard Western diet, your first step is to cut out eggs and dairy.

Thanks to the rise of veganism, these foods are easy to replace. So this is a great place to begin. There is no cooking to adapt here, the only thing you need to do is change the aisle you walk down in the supermarket. Instead of heading to the dairy aisle, just head to the plant milk aisle. Simple! If you are really lucky, like me, you might even be able to get fresh oat milk delivered to your doorstep–it's worth checking.

MILK (OR "LIQUID MEAT" AS IT IS SOMETIMES CALLED!)
Ten years ago, you would have struggled to find a good alternative to cow milk, even in large supermarkets. It still bogles my mind that we don't question a massive industry that is essentially ferrying the body fluids of a new mother to our doors! Luckily, these days, you are spoiled for choice–you have oat, soy, almond, hazelnut, cashew, coconut, and even milk made from peas or potatoes!

The great thing here is that instead of being stuck with one type of milk (cow milk) for your tea, coffee, smoothies or cereal, you can now enjoy a wide selection of different flavors. For example, hazelnut milk works beautifully with coffee, pea milk adds a nice amount of protein to your smoothies, and almond milk adds nuttiness to your morning muesli (my personal favorite!).

CHEESE
This one is commonly quoted as the reason people can't possibly go vegan. But now there are many new and exciting vegan cheeses to try–both from big brands like Violife and smaller artisan vegan cheesemakers that are popping up all over the place to answer this need we have for cheesy goodness. You can also easily make your own simple herby vegan cheese (and I've included the recipe below).

Thanks to @strictlyrootsvegan

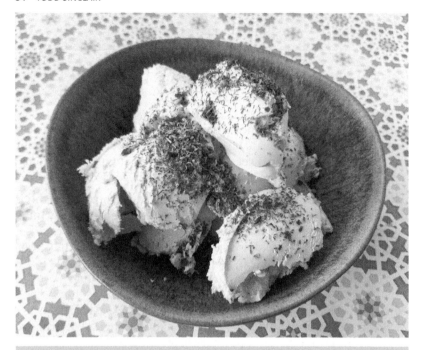

QUICK AND EASY VEGAN HERBY CASHEW SOFT CHEESE

INGREDIENTS:
- 1 cup cashew nuts (soaked overnight).
- 2 probiotic capsules (lactobacillus).
- 1 tsp Italian herb mix (or herbes de Provence).
- 1/8 tsp garlic granules (optional).
- Pinch of salt.

METHOD:
- Drain the cashews and place them in your high-speed blender. Blend until smooth. You might need to add a little water - try to add as little as possible because you want the mixture to stay quite thick (cream cheese consistency).
- Add the contents of two probiotic capsules and mix them in.
- Spoon the mixture into a bowl, cover it, and place in a warm dark place for 24 hours (for example an airing cupboard).
- When you check your mixture the next day, it should be aerated and smell slightly sour. If it isn't, leave it for another 24 hours.
- Mix in the herbs, garlic granules and salt.
- Spoon into a jar and store in the fridge. It will keep for 1 week.
- Spread on crackers, sandwiches, or use as a veggie dip.

HOW TO CHOOSE THE BEST PLANT-BASED DAIRY

Just like their dairy-based versions, some plant-based yogurts, cheeses and milk are basically just junk food: they are heavily processed and contain added sugar, preservatives and thickeners. A good place to start is to choose organic products, as these often contain fewer artificial ingredients and are less processed.

INGREDIENTS TO WATCH OUT FOR AND AVOID ARE:

- Sugar and other added sweeteners such as agave syrup, corn syrup, fructose, or sucrose. It's healthier to go for unsweetened yogurt and then add your own twist (for example fruit, dried fruit, oats, muesli, etc.)
- Thickeners are used to create the right yogurt consistency. But they are not created equal. Thickeners such as xanthan gum, guar gum, pectin and plant-based lecithin are safe. However, thickeners such as cellulose gum (carboxymethylcellulose), carrageenan, and polysorbate 80 can trigger digestive problems and are therefore best avoided.
- Additives such as titanium dioxide are sometimes added to make yogurt whiter. While it is generally recognized as safe by the FDA, I don't know how happy you feel about eating something that is also added to cosmetics and paint.
- Natural flavorings can also include unnatural flavorings made with chemicals, solvents, and preservatives. Go for unsweetened, unflavored vegan yogurt–you'll have a healthier starting point and can choose your own flavors to add.[1]

EGGS

Depending on how heavily eggs feature in your diet, you can cut them out here or wait until Week 4 when we eliminate all meat. There are plenty of great egg replacements available for recipes that traditionally call for eggs, or you can swap them for chia or flax eggs (simply mix 1 tablespoon of chia or flax with 3 tablespoons of warm water and voila–you have a healthy egg alternative).

If you enjoy baking, then research vegan recipes for your favorite cakes. I guarantee you will find several that can recreate your favorite baked goods without the animal products. Once you start veganizing, you'll be hooked.

YOGURT

If yogurt is an important part of your diet, you can swap it for coconut, almond, or soy-based yogurts instead. You can even make your own (you'll find a recipe for this below).

VEGAN YOGURT RECIPE
(INSPIRED BY THE FOOD REVOLUTION NETWORK)

INGREDIENTS:
- 2 cups cashews (soaked overnight)
- 2 tsp organic raw apple cider vinegar
- 1 cup water
- 1 pinch of salt (optional)
- 2 capsules of probiotic supplement (lactobacillus works well)

METHOD:
- Rinse and drain the cashew nuts, then place in a blender along with all the other ingredients, except the probiotic supplements.
- Blend until completely smooth and creamy (depending on your blender this will take between 1 and 4 minutes).
- Open the probiotic capsules and stir the powder into the blended cashews - use a wooden spoon or silicone spatula (metal spoons can stop the good bacteria from developing).
- Pour your cashew mix into a clean glass jar or bowl, and cover with a cheesecloth or clean and dry paper towel; use an elastic band to keep it in place and leave it somewhere safe.
- Wait 24-48 hours for the magic to happen. Taste the mix after 24 hours - if the flavor is slightly tangy, like yogurt, it's ready. If not, leave it for another 24 hours.
- Store your homemade vegan yogurt in the fridge and consume it within 5 days. You can also freeze it for up to a month.

OTHER OPTIONS:
- You can use a vegan yogurt starter - these are available in most health food shops. Simply follow the instructions.
- You can use 4 tablespoons of plain, unsweetened, organic vegan yogurt (simply mix this into the cashews once they are blended up).

ACTION PLAN FOR WEEK 1:

 Make your breakfasts plant-based. (See the Breakfast section of the Rebel Recipes for inspiration.)

 Invest in a good quality B12 supplement.

 Invest in a good quality vegan vitamin D supplement.

 Invest in a good quality vegan multivitamin.

 Explore new aisles: head to the supermarket and fill your trolley with plant-based goodies. Try a few types to find one you enjoy. Remember to check the label and focus on milk and yogurts that contain no added sugar, preservatives, artificial flavorings or colors.

 Embrace the new: change up your routine by trying out a new health food shop, buying an exotic fruit or unfamiliar vegetable and googling how to use it.

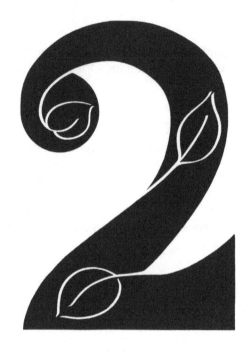

WEEK 2
THE FLEXITARIAN STAGE

The second step is to move to a flexitarian diet and cut out red meat. Also this week, your goal is to make both your breakfasts and lunches 100% plant-based. You can still have poultry and/or fish for dinner. This step might seem a little scary, but it's also exciting: you can begin exploring all the tasty vegan options on offer. When I first tasted a Beyond Burger, I knew I could be a full-time vegan!

ACTION PLAN FOR WEEK 2:

 Make both your breakfast and lunch 100% plant-based. There is a whole section of lunch recipes in Chapter 9.

 Find your tribe! One of the main reasons ex-vegans fall off the wagon is because they feel isolated and unsupported.1 Don't let this happen to you. There are plenty of great support networks out there, from Facebook groups to blogs. Join a local network and make some new plant-based buddies. Take a look at the Resource section at the end of the book for a list of good places to start.

 If you enjoy cooking, this is the time to invest in a good vegan cookbook (or more!) and start having some fun in the kitchen—after all, it is likely you've been stuck in a rut and eating the same foods day in and day out. This is your opportunity to rethink your dishes and start enjoying food all over again.

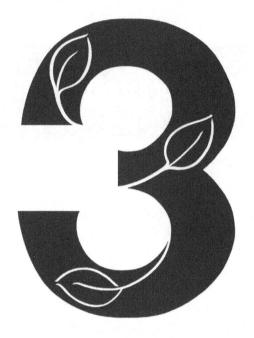

WEEK 3
DINNER - DOING THE PESCETARIAN

The third step is to go pescetarian. Cut out all land animals from your diet and begin making your dinners plant-based. Here, you can still "fall back" on seafood, but you should be revelling in your ongoing transformation and begin feeling healthier. Having massively reduced your consumption of animal products, your blood will be flowing better and your heart will be under less stress.[2] It's good to take stock and recognise your progression, improved health, and pat yourself on the back for coming this far.

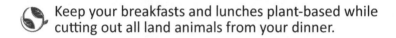

ACTION PLAN FOR WEEK 3:

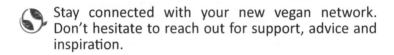 Keep your breakfasts and lunches plant-based while cutting out all land animals from your dinner.

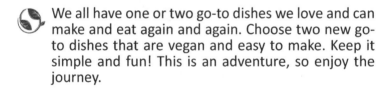 Stay connected with your new vegan network. Don't hesitate to reach out for support, advice and inspiration.

We all have one or two go-to dishes we love and can make and eat again and again. Choose two new go-to dishes that are vegan and easy to make. Keep it simple and fun! This is an adventure, so enjoy the journey.

Stay motivated by reviewing your key driving forces for change. You can also reach out to your support network for recognition of how far you've come.

If one of your driving forces is better health, this is a good time to check your blood pressure or jump on the scales - the results will incentivize you to keep going.

If you are feeling shaky, review your driving forces from Chapter 1 and my tips to staying motivated and inspired later in Chapter 7

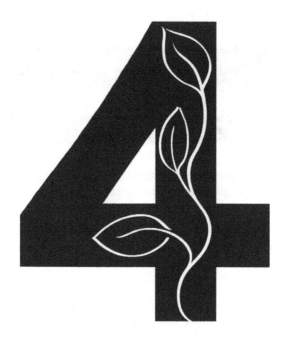

WEEK 4
MY NEW REALITY: COMING OUT

It's time to go fully plant-based! Cut out any remaining or lingering animal products from your diet. And if you didn't cut out eggs in Step I, now is the time to do it. Your blood will be flowing at its best since you were a baby. Hopefully—like a dog let off a lead—you are eager and motivated to start your new healthy life.

Congratulate yourself and share the news with your vegan tribe and support networks. Tune into yourself: how are you feeling–physically and emotionally–now you've gone through these steps? Do you feel ready to come out into the world as a new vegan? Are you feeling lighter, do you have more energy, have you lost some weight? This is the week you can start resting easier knowing that you are living a cruelty-free life, making a difference to climate change, and improving your longevity.

ACTION PLAN FOR WEEK 4:

 Veganize and make all meals & snacks 100% plant-based!

 Try some of the easy dinner recipes at the back of the book.

 Research local plant-based-friendly restaurants, cafés, and communities.

 If you feel ready, now is the time to come out to close family and friends. Share your news with the people you trust. There is no need to be smug here - your glowing health and enthusiasm should be shared and will be celebrated by anyone who loves you.

 Gratitude and self-care: you are making brave choices so pat yourself on the back and be good to yourself!

 Coming out party! Mark this achievement with a special treat or a night out. I have included my favorite curry and desert in the Rebel Cookbook at the end of this book. Or you can celebrate at your newfound local vegan restaurant!

 And as an extra reward to celebrate your new life, I've included my two favourite vegan chocolate recipes on the next page. Go treat yourself! Congratulations!

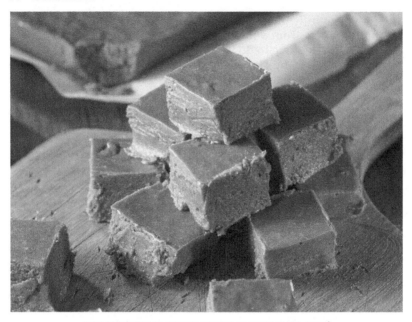

MAKE YOUR OWN VEGAN CHOCOLATE!
(2-INGREDIENT PEANUT CHOCOLATE FUDGE)

INGREDIENTS:
- 100g dark chocolate (choose an organic brand made with at least 75% cacao)
- 100g peanut butter (choose a brand made with peanuts and nothing else added)

METHOD:
- Chop the dark chocolate into small pieces, and place these in a bowl.
- Melt the chocolate over a bain-marie (place the bowl over a saucepan of boiling water).
- Once melted, add the peanut butter and mix until everything is combined.
- Pour into silicon molds or a container lined with parchment paper, and place in the fridge for an hour to set.
- Once set, store in an airtight container in the fridge. This will keep for at least 2 weeks (but mine never lasts that long!).
- Voila - easy healthy chocolate peanut fudge you can grab whenever you get a craving for something sweet.

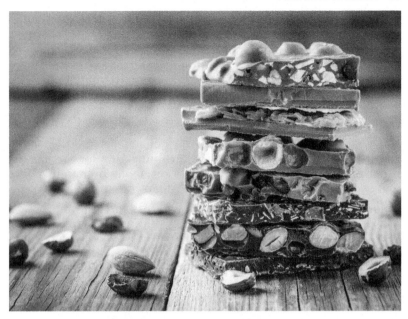

EASY ALMOND CHOCOLATE BITES

INGREDIENTS:
- 100g dark chocolate (choose an organic brand made with at least 75% cacao)
- 30g almond butter (choose a brand made with almonds and nothing else added)
- 50g roasted almonds (roughly chopped)
- Pinch of salt

METHOD:
- Chop the dark chocolate into small pieces, and place these in a bowl.
- Melt the chocolate over a bain-marie (place the bowl over a saucepan of boiling water).
- Once melted, add the almond butter and roasted almonds and mix until everything is combined.
- Pour into silicone molds or a container lined with parchment paper. Sprinkle it with salt and place in the fridge to set for an hour.
- Once set, store in an airtight container in the fridge.
- You can also get creative and use hazelnut butter and hazelnuts, or add granola instead of roasted nuts.

STAYING MINDFUL THROUGHOUT THIS JOURNEY

As you move along these steps, stay in touch with how you feel. By Week 4, you should notice quite a few changes. For one, you'll feel healthier. Most people lose unwanted weight and experience a surge in energy, as well as improved digestion. If you are diabetic, you should notice that your blood sugar levels are getting better. Although it is less noticeable, the same will be true for your cholesterol levels and blood pressure.

You will also notice that your cravings change. As you eat more whole, plant-based foods, you will start hungering for the healthy over the harmful. The more you choose vegetables over animals, the more your tastebuds will adapt and begin to crave those foods.

This is why I advise you to stick to the process and give your body a proper chance to adapt and give this new lifestyle time to transform you. This is like a new superpower you never knew you could harness. Allow yourself to be excited by this adventure and the power you have to create a better future–not just for yourself but for animals and for the planet. It truly is life-changing in every aspect. I am proud of you and thrilled to welcome you as a *REBEL VEGAN*!

WHAT TO DO ABOUT WITHDRAWAL SYMPTOMS?

We have all heard of withdrawal symptoms from things like caffeine, but did you know that you can get the same issue when you move away from the standard Western diet? A study published in the journal *Appetite* found that people who cut down on processed foods experience the same types of withdrawal symptoms as people who are addicted to drugs: sadness, tiredness, cravings, as well as increased irritability.[3]

This is hardly surprising when we remember that processed foods are packed with ingredients that hyper-stimulate the body—just like drugs, sugar and fat trigger a dopamine release that makes us feel good. This is why we turn to these foods again and again, especially when we need a lift. Whatever the guilty pleasure (whether it's French fries, pizza, donuts, or burgers), as we move away from these foods we have to find new ways to give ourselves the pleasure we crave.

According to the study, withdrawal symptoms lasted between two and five days, after which they cooled down somewhat. So the key thing to remember is that while you may experience cravings, it gets easier. You just have to stick with it. Another great way to navigate this is to plan ahead and have some fall-back foods ready in case a craving hits you.

Make a list of your guilty-pleasure foods and a counter-list of vegan versions that offer you the same flavor and texture experience without the addictive ingredients. Here are a few examples to get you started:

PROCESSED FOODS / ANIMAL PRODUCTS	PLANT-BASED ALTERNATIVES
Processed meats (ham, corned beef, chicken nuggets, burgers, sausages, etc.)	Marinated tofu or tempeh Seitan (avoid this if you are sensitive to gluten) Soy chunks Bean burgers or plant-based burgers Quorn or soy sausages
Ice-cream	Vegan ice-cream made from cashews, coconut, almond or soy Blended frozen banana (quickest, easiest ice-cream EVER)
Milkshakes	Peanut butter, banana and cacao smoothie Blueberry, banana, almond milk smoothie Mango, banana, coconut milk smoothie If you have a blender, there are no limits!
Supermarket bread	Home-made bread or bread from an independent local bakery, made with whole grains.
Sugary breakfast cereal	Granola made with oats, nuts, seeds, coconut, and dried fruit Overnight oats Porridge topped with coconut yogurt and fruit
Cookies, biscuits, cakes, pastries	Home-made energy balls (a mix of dried fruits, oats, nuts and seeds) Home-made vegan and refined-sugar-free cookies Home-made trail mix (for example with toasted almonds or cashews, pumpkin seeds, dried blueberries and cacao nibs)
Chocolate bars	Organic dark chocolate (at least 70%) Fruit & nut bars (choose brands made with no added flavors or sugar) Home-made vegan refined-sugar-free brownie
Crisps / chips	Kale crisps (simply mix kale with cashews and nutritional yeast and roast) Rice cakes or oat crackers with peanut butter Vegetable crisps (beetroot, carrot, zucchini, parsnip...)
Energy drinks and fizzy drinks	Green tea or herbal tea Kombucha Coconut water Sparkling water with a squeeze of lemon, crushed berries, or fresh mint
Pizza	Sourdough pizza with vegan cheese Home-made pizza on a sprouted grain tortilla Quick toastie with melted vegan cheese and sun-dried tomatoes and olives

It is easy to be a junk-food vegan–you can now find all your favorite ready meals and guilty-pleasures in plant-based form. While they don't contain animal-derived ingredients, these foods are as potentially harmful to your health as traditional processed foods. Having said that, they can be useful as you transition. What's more, I don't believe in denying yourself pleasure, that's why I'm a big fan of the 80-20 rule. This gives you some room for maneuver, particularly the first few weeks when you are navigating a new way of eating.

You will be surprised, once you begin, at just how easy it can be to move towards a diet where you're eating mostly whole plant-based foods that you prepare at home. This was part of the journey that I enjoyed the most: exploring new vegan foods and finding new recipes to try. Cooking new foods really opened up my world. Let it do the same for you.

YOUR VEGAN JOURNEY, YOUR RULES

The vegan movement is one of the fastest growing social justice movements in the world today.
DR. MELANIE JOY

It is your journey, and yours to design in a way that works for you. From Meatless Mondays to "mostly vegan," it is up to you to design and align your diet to fit your values.

As much as I would love to see the whole world go vegan overnight, I accept that it is overly ambitious to expect everyone to adopt a plant-based diet instantly. Food is so intrinsically tied in with culture, traditions and habits that it is more realistic to accept everyone's unique path and inspire by example.

I have never felt better, more confident and stronger, then when I gave up meat and diary. And there is a beautiful sense of peace when you embrace a life that is in line with your values. I believe all of us has the power to make a huge difference just by opening ourselves up to a more plant-based diet and cruelty-free life.

Taking things one meal at a time, we can change the world. I celebrate you for being here and being part in this global shift towards a more compassionate way of living.

YOU DON'T HAVE TO BE VEGAN EVERY DAY
But every day you are, on average you save:

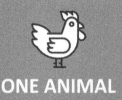

ONE ANIMAL

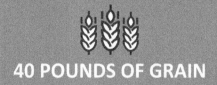

40 POUNDS OF GRAIN

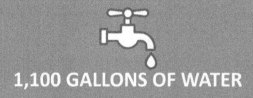

1,100 GALLONS OF WATER

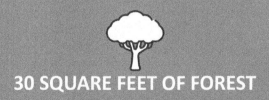

30 SQUARE FEET OF FOREST

Together, all those "every days"
start to add up to a massive change

FOR US, FOR ANIMAL WELFARE,
AND FOR THE PLANET

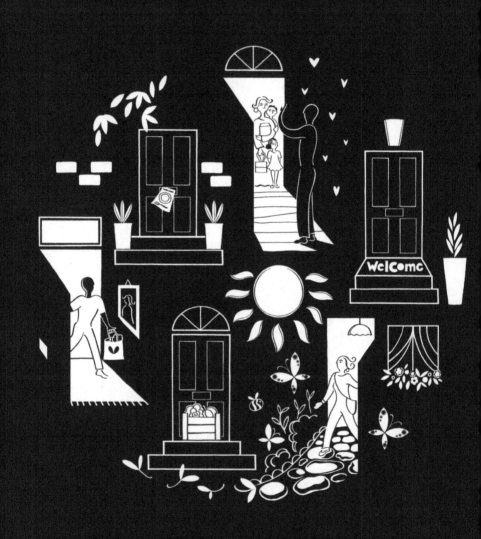

5

EATING IN, EATING OUT, COMING OUT

*"Living your best life is your most important
journey in life."*
OPRAH WINFREY

Creating and maintaining a plant-powered life has its challenges, but it is also a great adventure that will bring huge rewards. This chapter is all about navigating that journey. Here are my practical guidelines and tips to help you implement a plant-based diet as effortlessly as possible.

EATING IN

PARTY IN MY PLANT-BASED KITCHEN!

BUDGET AND BULK-BUYING:

Many new vegans find that they actually save money on food bills, despite the often-mentioned argument that eating a healthier diet is more expensive. The great thing about a plant-based diet is that many staples are easy to stock and can be bought in bulk every month or so: canned tomatoes, beans, lentils, whole grains (rice, whole grain pasta, bean noodles, buckwheat noodles.) coconut milk, nuts, seeds, flour, spices, and dried herbs. Then all you need to do is buy fresh vegetables and fruits every week to create delicious, nutritious meals.

READING THE LABELS:

Many food companies proudly advertise their vegan products. Simply look for the little "V" mark that indicates the food is completely plant-based. If this mark is not present, it's about reading the label. You'll find a link to my favorite food label guide in the Resources section. While some foods are easy to identify as vegan (because of the "V" symbol), many foods you might think would be vegan actually contain milk, honey, eggs or gelatin–and you'll only find that out if you read the label.

NAVIGATING A NEW SHOPPING EXPERIENCE:

Shopping will feel different, especially in the beginning. You may need to give yourself more time to navigate aisles you've not walked down, and to read labels. Once you get comfortable with the products and brands you can trust, this will become much easier, but you'll still have to stay aware.

Get yourself online and look for recommendations by other vegans, for example foods known as "accidentally vegan." These are foods that weren't intended to be vegan, but don't contain any animal ingredients. A well-known example is Oreo cookies.

NAVIGATING A NEW COOKING EXPERIENCE:

A great way to learn how to structure your meals is to try vegan meal kits, such as those delivered by Purple Carrot, Daily Harvest, or Veestro (there are many more![1]). Each kit is a complete meal containing all the macro-nutrients you need. I didn't just learn some tasty recipes (the Purple Carrot burger is the best I've ever had), but also how to design nutritious meals. These kits can help you get into the rhythm and discover new dishes. An old-fashioned cookbook is also highly recommended!

A WELL-STOCKED PANTRY:

Give your kitchen cupboards a vegan make-over!

As you use up all the old packs of processed foods and animal products, you can begin restocking your pantry to make plant-based eating effortless. The trick here is to ensure you have all the ingredients you need to throw together vegan meals, simply with the addition of a few fresh vegetables or fruits.

Here is a snapshot of my pantry, to inspire you to create your own, based on the recipes you enjoy cooking. You don't have to have all these ingredients (indeed, stocking ten varieties of plant milk might be going a little over the top), but this table gives you an idea of what you need to start cooking healthy, tasty, easy vegan meals.

TODD'S PANTRY LIST

WHOLE GRAINS	BEANS & LÉGUMES	OILS & SEASONINGS	BAKING & HEALTHY TREATS
Rice (brown rice, Venus black rice, wild rice) Buckwheat Quinoa Millet Polenta Oats Oat crackers Pasta or noodles made from brown rice, whole grain spelt, whole grain wheat, or buckwheat	You can buy canned for convenience and speed - make sure you choose brands with only beans and water, nothing else added) Chickpeas Black beans Kidney beans Cannellini beans Black eye beans Borlotti beans Mung beans (Adzuki beans Lentils (green or red) Split peas	Olive oil Coconut oil Avocado oil Sesame oil Flax oil Olives Sun-dried tomatoes Vegan mayonnaise Tamari sauce or soy sauce Apple cider vinegar Himalayan salt or other natural & unrefined salt Nutritional yeast	Whole grain spelt flour Whole grain wheat flour Rice flour Buckwheat flour Coconut flour Ground almonds Egg replacer Baking powder Vanilla essence or powder Dates Apricots Raisins Maple syrup, rice syrup, or vegan honey Cacao powder

SPICES & HERBS	NUTS & SEEDS	MILK & DAIRY ALTERNATIVES	CANNED GOODS
Cinnamon Turmeric Cumin Coriander Garam masala Ras el Hanout Italian herb mix or Herbes de Provence Mild curry powder Smoked paprika Oregano Rosemary Fennel seed Black pepper	Tahini Peanut butter Almond butter Cashew butter Hazelnut butter Pumpkin seeds Sunflower seeds Chia seeds Flax seeds Sesame seeds Hemp seeds Almonds Hazelnuts Cashew nuts Brazil nuts Coconut flakes or desiccated coconut Pine nuts	Almond milk Soy milk Oat milk Cashew milk Pea milk Hazelnut milk Tiger nut milk Silken tofu Soy cream Oat cream Almond cream Probiotic capsules or vegan starters (if you want to make your own vegan yogurt or cheese)	Canned tomatoes Canned jackfruit Canned coconut milk Canned beans (see beans & legumes)

FROM VEGAN READY-MEALS TO VEGAN HOME-COOKING:
The best advice I can offer here is to start small and build from that.

Before you began your 4-week journey to veganism, you sat down with your schedule and worked out when you have free time and when you have spare energy–these are the moments you can dedicate to meal planning and meal prepping.

For example, say you have some spare time and energy on Sunday afternoon. You could spend a few hours getting food ready for the week. For example, by making a hearty pasta-bake or a big pot of curry, which can easily be portioned and frozen for later–then what you basically have is a ready-meal which contains only healthy ingredients, but is just as convenient and quick as supermarket meals. Meal prep does not have to be complicated–you just have to double, triple, or quadruple your ingredients, and voila! You've got ready-made food for the week.

It is also easy to batch-prepare things like chia puddings, energy balls, roasted nuts –all of which make tasty snacks. If you are taking lunches to work, you could prepare salad jars for a few days simply by cooking up a load of rice or other grains, and then layering the rice with beans and chopped vegetables (carrots, celery, radish, zucchini, sweet peppers, kale, etc.) in jars, and storing in the fridge.

You can also make hummus and salad dressings, which keep for about a week, and mean you'll always have something tasty to dip vegetables into or use as a sandwich spread. Once you start this process, you'll feel into the best method for your unique circumstances–whether you live on your own, work from home, or cook for your family.

As you begin, go easy on yourself. If you have to fall back on a vegan ready-meal every so often, that is okay. Remember the 80-20 rule. It's not about aiming for perfection, it's about creating a lifestyle you can sustain for the long term.

The more you cook from scratch, the more instinctive it will feel. You do not need to be a Masterchef candidate, nor spend hours in the kitchen to prepare tasty food. A well-stocked vegan pantry and a little bit of planning is all you need.

MAKE SURE YOU EAT ENOUGH AND EAT WHAT YOU LOVE:
If you feel hungry or are uninspired by what you're eating, then you will fall off the vegan wagon. That's why it is so important that you eat filling and flavorful food. When you are full and satiated, it is much easier to say no to temptations.

FIND YOUR FAVORITE VEGAN ALTERNATIVES:

Take the time to search for plant-based substitutes to your favorite animal products. You can make this a fun experience by buying several brands and then having a taste-test (maybe with some fellow vegan newbies, or curious friends). Gone are the days when there was just one option (soy milk!). These days most supermarkets stock at least three types of vegan cheese, countless plant milk varieties, not to mention vegan burgers.

BE THE FRIENDLY VEGAN IN YOUR SHARED HOUSE:

If you live in a house-share, changing your diet can feel daunting, but it doesn't have to be. It is usually easy to compartmentalize the kitchen and fridge space so that your shelves are kept vegan. Sit your roommates down and let them know you are making this change. Reassure them that you are not about to become "one of those vegans" who judge others for their choices, and that you're not going to bombard them with stats and facts while they're trying to enjoy their burger. This way, you will ensure there is no animosity in the household. After all, living together is an art form. The best thing you can do for the vegan movement is be kind and compassionate with others–they are on their own path!

CHOOSE MEALS YOU CAN EASILY ADAPT FOR YOUR NON-VEGAN LOVED ONES:

If you need to juggle different diets in your household, family, or relationship, this can be challenging. After all, meals are there to be shared. The easiest way to navigate this is to make meals that can be easily added to.

For example, you can prepare the joint meal in an assembly line style, and add the meat at the end. You can prepare the chicken/seafood/mince separately and add it at the last minute to the plate, stir-fry, curry, stew or casserole. As a rule, the defining flavor of a dish is the sauce, so you can experience and enjoy the meal together.

TAKE IT SLOW WITH BEANS, PEAS, AND LENTILS:

As you adapt from a diet high in saturated fats and animal products to a plant-based diet that contains a lot more fiber, you might find you get a bit too gassy. If this happens, it is a sign you need to give your body a little time to adapt to new foods.

As a general rule, beans and pulses are the main culprits when it comes to bloating and gas. The bloating comes from the indigestible fibers in the beans' shell. These become easier to digest if you soak the beans overnight and cook them thoroughly. Staying in tune with your body will help too—try different beans and lentils to see which ones you tolerate better, and go slowly.

EATING OUT: LET'S MAKE IT FUN!

*You are only confined by the walls
that you build yourself*
REBEL VEGAN

Eating out is never just about the food. It's a social occasion, a way to catch up with friends and family, a moment we savor because we have our loved ones around us AND we won't need to do the washing up (win-win!). However, if your friends and family are meat-eaters, you might feel awkward asking about plant-based options. But fear not! These days, so many restaurants and cafes serve vegan options, and even those that don't have vegan options on the menu will help you out if you call ahead.

Better still, there's an app for that! Both *Happy Cow* and *Vanilla Bean* allow you to search by location, or use GPS to show you all the places near you that are either vegan or serve vegan options. It's time to challenge (if you feel comfortable to) and inspire your loved ones to try something new.

MY EATING OUT TIPS:
- **Get the apps:** *Happy Cow* is your best friend when it comes to exploring vegan-friendly eateries. You might be surprised at how many options there are locally.
- **Plan ahead:** If it's an organized event, you can contact the restaurant (by phone, WhatsApp or Facebook Messenger), get a copy of the menu, check the vegan options, and ask questions. With a little charm, it is usually easy to develop a rapport, and most restaurants will fall over themselves to be helpful. That way you can avoid any anxiety, just relax and enjoy the occasion.
- **Prepare for social events:** Most hosts are mindful and ask about dietary requirements, allergies, and likes or dislikes when they send out their invitation. Be polite but honest - the worst thing you can do is not tell a host you're vegan. You can also offer to bring food if you feel this would put the host under undue stress. Most hosts will refuse that offer and work with you to find a solution. If the event is a potluck dinner, bring your favorite vegan party food and share it with other guests (this is a great opportunity to showcase just how delicious plant-based food can be!). If you know there will be no vegan options at the event, eat a large meal beforehand and take some snacks with you.
- **Practice makes perfect:** If it's an impromptu event and you haven't had time to organize in advance, don't worry. With a little practice, you will soon be able to scan a menu and see what can be eaten or adapted. Until then, just fake it 'til you make it: turn on the charm and ask the waiter which dish can be made vegan. Don't be timid—you are a *REBEL VEGAN*! Be confident and comfortable. There's usually one or two dishes that can easily be modified to be vegan. Stir-fries are easily adaptable (for example, by removing chicken or prawns).

- **Ask for the secret menu:** Did you know that some restaurants have secret menus? Just ask. Often there is a vegetarian or vegan menu stashed away somewhere.

- **Get creative with side dishes:** A few sides of brown rice, beans and vegetables quickly add up to a balanced meal. Learn to laugh and pretend it's a tapas night.

- **Flirt:** Yes, a little gentle flirtation with the waiting staff will have them eating out of your hand. With the waiter on side, you'll be able to figure out some vegan options together.

- **Carry snacks:** If you think the options will be severely limited, then eat beforehand and/or during.

- **Go international.** Ethnic cuisines usually have the best plant-based traditions and options. Indian, Thai, Vietnamese, Mexican, or Mediterranean restaurants traditionally have many plant-based options.

- **Don't sweat the small stuff:** It might seem a challenge at first, but in the scheme of things it is only a meal. Focus on the occasion and the people, rather than the food.

- **Leave a review:** Especially if the restaurant has been super helpful. This is how we spread this compassionate revolution!

- **On the bright side, most alcohol is vegan.** But if you want to be sure, you can use the *Barnivore* website (you'll find the link in the resources section) to check whether your wine is vegan-friendly (some wines are filtered using animal products).

The main thing to remember is to be kind to yourself! Being vegan is not a competition. You're not going to be disqualified if you accidentally-on-purpose eat cheese or accept a slice of your grandmother's pumpkin pie! *REBEL VEGANS* make–and break–the rules, but always strive for compassion and justice.

VEGAN ON-THE-GO AND TRAVELING VEGAN - SNACK IDEAS:

- Peanut butter sandwiches (and the innumerable varieties: such as peanut butter and jelly, peanut butter and banana, peanut butter and chocolate spread...)

- Fruit and nut mixes: you can buy these ready-made or prepare your own at home (for example by roasting almonds, cashews, walnuts, pumpkin seeds, and adding dates, cranberries, raisins, coconut flakes, cacao nibs...)

- Hummus: it's easy to carry a little Tupperware of Hummus, bean dip, or guacamole you can eat with rice cakes or vegetable sticks.

- Granola bars: another very transportable snack. Here again, you can find good vegan granola bars or energy bars in most supermarkets (check the ingredient label and choose the ones made with whole foods only and no added sugar), or you can make some at home.

- For tips to stay vegan on the road, check out my *REBEL VEGAN* Travel Guide!

COMING OUT
SHOWING UP AS A *REBEL VEGAN*

"Accept who you are. Unless you're a serial killer."
ELLEN DEGENERES[2]

As a REBEL VEGAN, you will need to find your inner strength to come out to your friends, your family, and the world. While we are trailblazers in an important social movement, we are also very misunderstood and often discriminated against.[3] This is known as vegaphobia. Yes, it is a thing!

In 2015, a study published in the Journal Group Processes & Intergroup Relations entitled "It ain't easy eating greens" found that vegans and vegetarians in Western societies experience discrimination on a par with other minorities.[4]

However, unlike other forms of bias (such as racism or sexism), negativity towards people who choose to eat plants over animals is not considered a social problem. In fact, it is both commonplace, largely accepted as "normal", and often left unaddressed.[5]

Be ready to navigate this new world with grace and poise. Learn to build your armor around you. Very often people react negatively towards vegans because of their own unconscious discomfort with their diet. After all, eating meat requires a cognitive dissonance of some kind. It requires people to shut their eyes and ears to the atrocities committed by the meat industry to animals and the planet.

When you show up as a REBEL VEGAN, you shine a light on other people's choices, and this can be uncomfortable for them. So, remember to smile and leave judgment at the door–just because they are judging your choices, does not mean you have to judge theirs. Remind them that your diet choices do not directly affect them–live and let live.

One of the big problems is this: you find yourself being lectured about why you "need" meat, usually by people who are not qualified nutritionists anyway. Or people will assume you're surviving on a diet of carrots, celery and lettuce. Naturally, you will want to explain yourself (Chapter 11 of this companion book *REBEL VEGAN: A New Take on Veganism For a Brave New World*, delves deeper into this, and looks at the most common anti-vegan arguments and how to answer them with confidence). But when you do, you risk being labeled as "that vegan" who "doesn't shut up about veganism." It's almost like you can't win. But let me assure you–going vegan means you are winning and you're on the right side of history.

If you are confronted by sarcasm, simply be gently assertive in return. Try not to get sucked into arguments. With time, you will learn to recognize when you can have a sensible conversation about the topic, or whether the person in front of you is simply lashing out. If the conversation takes a turn for the more aggressive, you can simply state your truth and change the subject.

Don't let other people's opinions of your lifestyle choices affect you. When people judge, it's less about you, more about them. Just keep your focus on the positive changes you're making. Ultimately, you are not responsible for changing people's minds. We can only lead by example and focus on being the best versions of ourselves.

In this book, I share my coming out story. And, within this book, you have the tools to build your own unique journey towards veganism. Along the way, you will also find your confidence to come out and be a proud vegan. By embracing your inner rebel, you are living authentically, aligned with your core ethics, and being the change you want to see in the world.

MY MANTRA
IF YOU CAN VISUALIZE IT, YOU CAN VEGANIZE IT.

VEGANISM ON THE ROAD: MY TRANSITION

When I went vegan, I was living and working on the road as an international tour manager in South East Asia. I would be living out of a suitcase for months at a time while taking groups through countries like Vietnam, Laos, Myanmar, and Cambodia. Some places were more accommodating than others. In Thailand, for example, there were bigger supermarkets where I could always stock up on vegan essentials - mine were almond milk and muesli. This way, I could always start my day with a plant-based meal and avoid the egg-based breakfasts that most hotels served. My bag was always heavy with plant-based staples. While crossing land borders with my heavy bags, I felt like an almond milk mule!

I learned to laugh at misunderstandings and enjoy eating sticky rice. I became pretty well known throughout South East Asia for taking over kitchens and street vendors and demonstrating first-hand what vegan cooking looked like.

After returning many times, I developed a bond with many restaurants in the region. I was trusted to go into the kitchen and help explain and cook vegan food with their staff. People in my groups would laugh and offer me a tip for cooking and delivering their food. A few of them jokingly called me the vegan Gordan Ramsey. But I like to think I was slightly more diplomatic!

After I ensured my group was fed, I would often stay and eat on the floor with my new friends in the kitchen. And I was continually surprised and impressed how the locals seemed to get veganism like second nature. It didn't cause as much tension as in the west and was instantly accepted as a perfectly logical lifestyle choice. They instinctively understood the philosophy of compassion, as it fits so seamlessly within their traditional values and Buddhist principles. They helped me realize my passion to veganize the world.

Veganism has opened up my world, never restricted it. I never saw it as a chore. Rather, it was a daily opportunity to engage with people and connect on a different level. Many were interested and receptive. The world is changing, and they want to be part of it. Some of my favorite moments were when I would return to these little towns and the owners would proudly present their new vegan menu with a wink. It felt like we were on the map.

Then, when I returned to the UK, I thought, how does this work? I remember walking down supermarket aisles I'd never noticed, searching for the "vegetarian" sign. There was a tiny section in the chilled meals section, and often only soy milk. But every time I returned to London, this section grew bigger. It was like coming back to a city under construction and witnessing the progress - new products, more options, a wider selection. Suddenly, all the supermarkets had their own plant-based range, and plant-based milks took over the health foods aisle. I still get excited each time I notice a new vegan range or product. It is my guilty pleasure to try them all. All in the name of research, of course!

My travels have always taken me back home to my vegan values that underpin everything I do. Veganism has given me the confidence and peace of mind to go out into the world as my authentic self. And this, in turn, has brought so many amazing people and places into my orbit. But there is no better feeling than coming home.

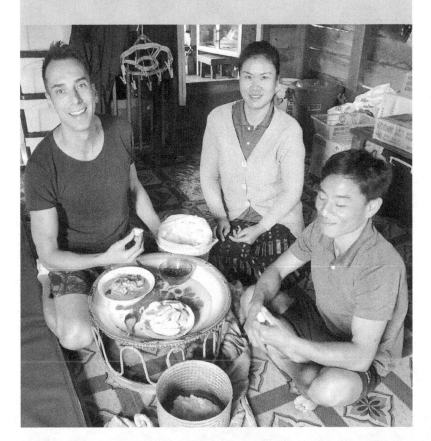

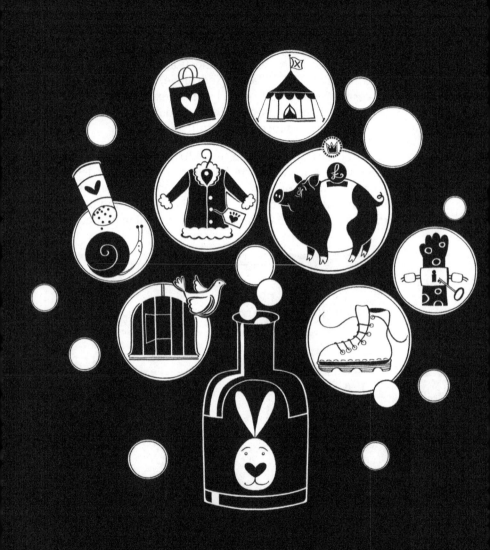

6

BEYOND DIET
VEGAN CHIC

"Traditional animal testing is expensive, time-consuming, uses a lot of animals and from a scientific perspective the results do not necessarily translate to humans."
DR. CHRISTOPHER AUSTIN,
FORMER DIRECTOR OF THE NATIONAL INSTITUTES OF HEALTH[1]

"The history of cancer research has been a history of curing cancer in the mouse. We have cured mice of cancer for decades and it simply didn't work in humans."
DR. RICHARD KLAUSNER,
FORMER DIRECTOR OF THE NATIONAL CANCER INSTITUTE[2]

What you have already braved and achieved is profound. I believe this knowledge is powerful, and we should use it wisely and ethically. We can transcend many of the global issues we face—species extinction, climate change, global pandemics, and disease epidemics—by going plant-based and cruelty-free. By transitioning to veganism, you have now lined up your beliefs and values with your lifestyle. Be happy and confident in your strong choices - you are making a positive impact on the world!

Now you have shifted your diet, you can explore other ways to build on your cruelty-free, sustainable life. Although I don't want to overwhelm you, I think it is important to consider the wider message of the vegan movement and use your awareness holistically.

A fully vegan lifestyle excludes all forms of exploitation and cruelty to animals, as far as practicable and possible. Diet is a huge part of that, but unfortunately animals are exploited in many other ways. Going fully vegan extends past dietary choices–iit includes not going to zoos, wearing wool or leather, nor using cosmetics and products tested on animals.

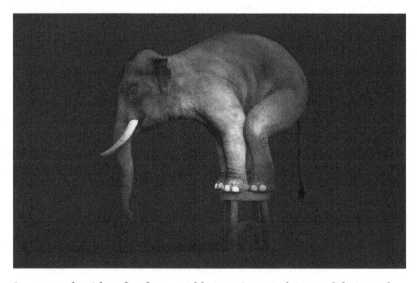

I grew up beside a fox farm and have witnessed, in my lifetime, that whole industry implode as the top fashion houses ditched fur, and we all rethink what luxury is.

As you move along the spectrum towards veganism, you will feel empowered by your positive changes. If you feel emboldened to do so, you can become an ethical vegan and create a fully plant-based lifestyle. Going all the way means no honey or leather shoes. It feels fantastic to know you are living a fully cruelty-free life. So let's cast off those final carnistic shackles!

As your awareness increases and you remove animal products from your shopping trolley and kitchen cupboards, this inevitably brings up questions and uncomfortable realities around what you buy and wear. At this point, you can start to rethink your entire lifestyle: how cruelty-free are your fashion choices? Have your toiletries been tested on animals? This involves doing a little research to check the small print on everything from labels to the ethos of your go-to brands.

Just to reiterate, this is an optional final step, food for thought, planting a seed. I commend and support where you are right now. Just by questioning and changing your diet, you have made one of the most effective and positive impacts on the world!

If you would like to take it further, here are my tips for taking your veganism to the next level.

TOILETRIES AND HOUSEHOLD PRODUCTS

The thing to look out for first is the little "V" mark, which indicates the product is certified vegan. This means it doesn't contain animal-derived ingredients, and has not been tested on animals. If the little "V" is not present on the product packaging, you will need to check the brand's website to see whether they are cruelty-free or not.

Another thing to consider is the secondary effects of these products. For example, we know that products containing microplastic, solvents, and chemicals, are flushed down the drain and end up in all our water supplies. Even if these products are vegan, they harm aquatic life and pollute our planet.

If you want to take things to the next level, start phasing out your current products by finding vegan and green alternatives. The good news is it is easier than ever to find non-toxic, cruelty-free toiletries, make-up, and household products. Just head to your local health food shop and browse the household product aisle.

FASHION

Fast fashion is the second most polluting industry worldwide. According to the United Nations Environment Program (UNEP), the fashion industry is the second largest polluter of water globally. Every second, the equivalent of one garbage truck of textile is either landfilled or burned. If things continue as they are, this industry will use up a quarter of the world's carbon budgets. Fast fashion also uses plastic-derived textiles (polyester, for example), which accounts for around 9% of the microplastics in the ocean.[3] It takes 2,700 liters (713 gallons) of water to make enough cotton for just one t-shirt.[4]

There is also a human cost to the fashion industry. Most of us have heard about sweatshops and the conditions textile workers are forced to endure (low wages, long hours, unsanitary and unsafe working conditions), just so we can buy that cheap t-shirt.

Last but not least, animals experience torture and a violent death for wool, leather, suede, feathers, and fur. None of this is necessary, especially now that fake fur and vegan leather are so widespread and relatively easy to find.

We have gotten used to disposable fashion, but we can move away from it. Going vegan does not mean you have to exist in beige slacks and forget about being fashionable–far from it! But it requires a rethink of where you buy and how often you buy new clothes.

Here are a few ideas to help you create your cruelty-free wardrobe:

- Go second-hand! You'll be surprised just how much fun this can be. The buzz you get when you find the perfect outfit for a few dollars/pounds/euros is well worth rummaging around for.
- Have a clothes swap evening. Gather your friends for a (vegan) pot-luck dinner and clothing exchange. Everyone brings a dish and a few unwanted clothes, and everyone leaves with a new item. One person's garbage is another's treasure.
- Ask your network for recommendations: there are many ethical, vegan, cruelty-free fashion brands out there. So ask around and explore different options. You might just be surprised at how fashionable it can be to be vegan!
- Choose wisely: vegan leather is wonderful, but what materials have been used instead? Are they recycled plastics or virgin plastics? Is the clothing retailer really ethical, or have they just simply launched a "green" collection to greenwash their image?

ETHICAL BRANDS

This is where a little research is necessary. But as your awareness grows, you'll be able to sense whether a brand is ethical or not. And with a little practice, you'll also see through the green-washing and whether those brands who have jumped on the vegan bandwagon as lip-service and marketing rather than real compassion.

An example would be those global fast food giants. Yes, they now offer vegan options. But are they making a positive difference to the world, or are their practices destroying the planet and harming animals? Have they added a vegan option to their menu because they care about improving the state of the world, or because they've spotted an opportunity for increased profits? Unfortunately, I would say it's the latter. I'm not saying you shouldn't eat there, but it is worth thinking about the impact of the corporations we buy from.

Here are some questions to consider when choosing your new go-to brands:

- Are they sustainable? In other words, do they use sustainable materials or ingredients? Do they consider their impact on the environment and society? For example, by choosing local, independent supply chains, reducing their greenhouse gas emissions, or setting up local charities.
- Are they transparent? A really ethical company will be transparent about where and how they source their raw materials, how they treat their staff, and whether they test their products on animals. If you contact the company and don't get answers, it's a good sign that their practices are not ethical. Companies that care about their impact will be proud to share this with you. Look for clear, specific, and well-organized information.
- Do they have third-party certifications to confirm their positive impact? These aren't always foolproof, but it is a good place to start. For example, the Fair-trade certification is designed to help producers in developing countries get a fair price for their products and achieve sustainable, equitable trade relationships, but this isn't always the case. A study published by MIT Press found that benefits to producers were negligible because of an oversupply of certifications.[5] There are also question marks around whether Fairtrade can enforce fair trade standards. But there are certain certifications you can trust. For example, Certified B Corporations, which aim to use business as a force for good, balance purpose and profit, and are legally required to consider their impact on workers, customers, suppliers, community, and the environment.[6]

GREENWASHING AND HUMANE-WASHING

Talking nice about sun and wind
and green jobs is just greenwash.
DR JAMES HANSEN, NASA SCIENTIST[7]

If something sounds a little too good to be true, it's usually worth digging a little deeper. Many brands use greenwashing to downplay their environmental impact and hoodwink consumers that their products are greener or less harmful than they truly are. When Shell or Exxonmobil launch adverts about their solar energy and wind turbines while staying silent about their more polluting practices (such as their plans to drill under the Arctic), this is greenwashing. Other strategies also include funding studies that mislead the public or confuse the climate change argument. Think of how the tobacco industry encouraged people to smoke by using doctors to recommend their products.

Humane-washing is similar to greenwashing. An increasingly desperate animal agriculture industry is using this new tactic to convince the public that their products are produced humanely, even as the evidence to the contrary becomes impossible to ignore. Cue images of well-fed, happy cows and cheeky chickens gently and lovingly herded by an attentive, friendly farmer. Most of the labels you will see on animal products, such as "free-range", "cage-free", "family-farmed", and "responsibly sourced", are deceptive (please see my companion book *REBEL VEGAN LIFE: A Radical Take on Veganism For a Brave New World* to find out more).

Similarly, the powerful farming industry funds studies to proclaim that meat and dairy are "proven" to be healthy, while denouncing a vegan diet as "deficient." Meanwhile, a mountain of well-documented evidence shows the exact opposite. They are using the same dirty tactics as the cigarette corporations and trying to confuse and keep us hooked.

I am the ultimate vegan realist. Whether it's green or humane-washing, these labels are not there to protect the environment nor the animals, but to mislead you into thinking you're buying something sustainable. It's a cover-up to try to muddy the waters. Therefore, we have to scrutinize these false narratives and see through the marketing. This way, we defend truth and justice.

A *REBEL VEGAN* needs to be able to recognise these deliberate distractions and see through these industry-driven studies and headlines about products that have been shown time and time again to be harmful to our health, animals, and the planet. These massive corporations have invested billions to mislead and convince the public they care. Therefore, we have to be vigilant and prepared to fight for justice and truth.

SPOTTING GREENWASHING AND HUMANE-WASHING:

- Does the brand's sustainability page answer your questions, or are you left with more questions than answers? If it's greenwashing/humane-washing, you'll just get lots of big statements and nice images, but nothing to back these claims up. If it's really ethical, you'll find information about their approach to materials, employees, emissions, and even what to do with their products once you've used them (for example, information on where to send old items for repair, donation, or recycling).

- Does the brand have any third-party certifications, and how do these certifications impact the brand's ethical and environmental responsibilities? Are the products themselves certified, or just the materials or factory used to make them?

- Who owns the brand? It is common for huge corporations with questionable ethics to buy independent brands or launch new brands under another name to conquer more of the market-place or attract eco-consumers. For example, Nestlé owns Haagen Dazs, Nespresso, and KitKat[8], while CocaCola owns Innocent Smoothies, and Honest Tea, among others.[9] You will usually find this information in the small print of their website.

- Check the small print: Who's funded the study? Do the researchers have any conflicts of interest? Are there studies that prove the exact opposite?

- Ultimately, beware of claims that sound too good to be true! Once you know what to look for, spotting greenwashing and humane-washing is pretty simple.

Once you're on the journey towards veganism and feel that increasing sense of contentment from being aligned with your ethics, it's not hard to build momentum.

Being a *REBEL VEGAN* starts with diet, but inevitably goes further. Even if you do not feel ready to make these changes now, you'll notice that the longer you are vegan, the more you will be attracted to brands that take their social, environmental, and ethical responsibilities seriously. As you shift towards a kinder diet, you will naturally want to shift to a kinder, more sustainable, and compassionate lifestyle.

This is how we create a better world.
One step at a time - it starts with you.

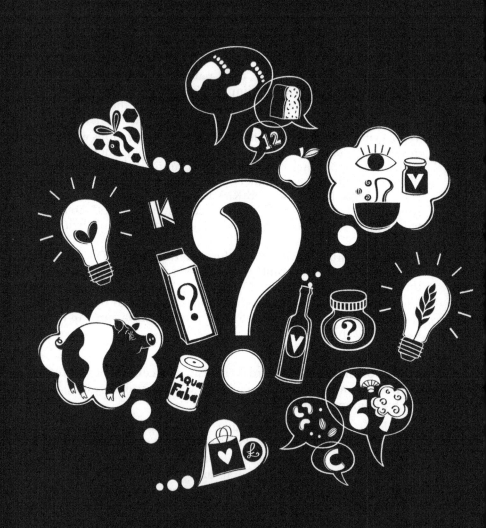

7

11 SECRETS TO STAY MOTIVATED

*Put your heart, mind, and soul
into even your smallest acts.*
SWAMI SIVANANDA[1]

*The true secret of happiness lies in taking a
genuine interest in all the details of daily life.*
WILLIAM MORRIS[2]

*The secret of your future is hidden in your daily
routine.*
MIKE MURDOCK[3]

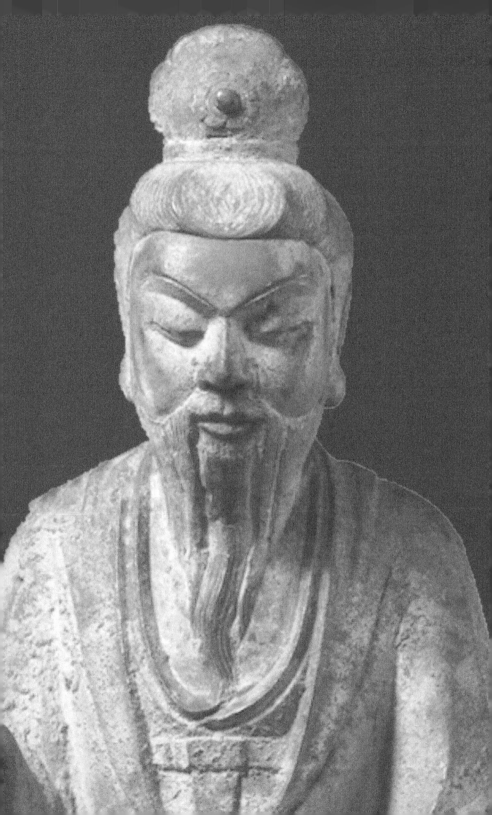

1. KEEP IT SUPER SIMPLE:

THE KISS PRINCIPLE

This is not about being a gourmet chef. If you overcomplicate your diet, or put too much pressure on yourself, you will likely become exasperated and give up. Focus on simple meals made with fresh ingredients. You're not practicing for MasterChef!

"Perfection is the enemy of progress."
WINSTON CHURCHILL[4]

"Simplicity, patience, compassion.
These three are your greatest treasures."
TAO TE CHING - LAO TZU[5]

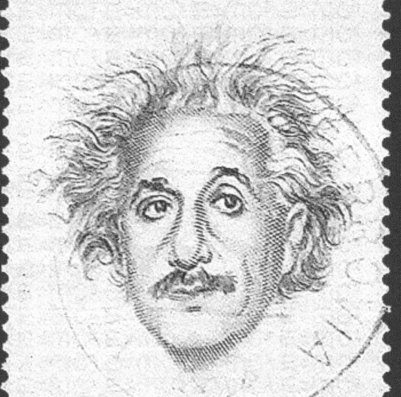

ALBERT EINSTEIN 1879-1955

ITALIA 120

I.P.Z.S.-ROMA-1979

F. TULLI

2. OPEN YOUR MIND:
EXPAND YOUR VISION PAST THE HERE AND NOW

Everything you might want is available in vegan form these days–
from cheese to sushi. Sure, it isn't 100% the same thing, but at least it
is in alignment with your ethics. Open your mind to new flavors and
experiences. I turned a corner when I discovered that plant-based
burgers taste much better than their animal-based counterparts.
I have learned to enjoy the adventure. And remember: your taste
buds will soon adjust!

*"Progress is impossible without change,
and those who cannot change their minds cannot
change anything."*
GEORGE BERNARD SHAW[6]

*"The mind that opens up to a new idea never
returns to its original size. The measure of
intelligence is the ability to change."*
ALBERT EINSTEIN[7]

"An open heart is an open mind."
DALAI LAMA[8]

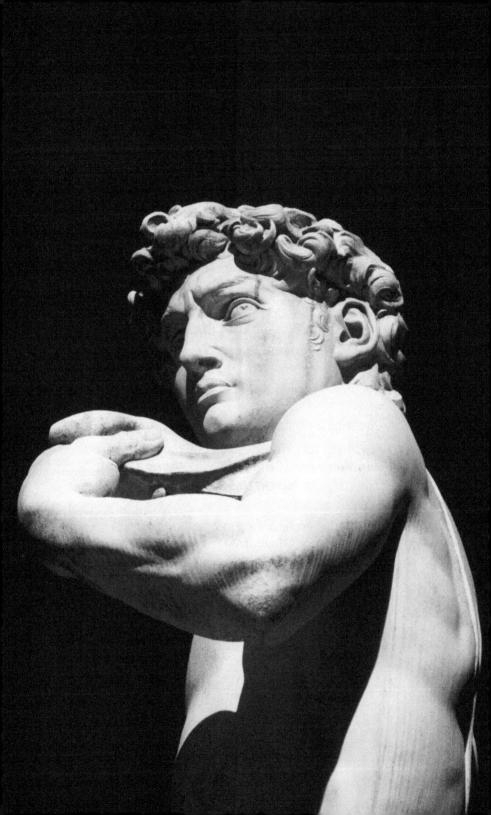

3. PATIENCE IS A VIRTUE:
BE PATIENT WITH YOUR TASTE BUDS

They have a short memory–cravings for meat will soon pass as you begin tasting different foods and healthier flavors. Keep the faith, as eating plants will soon become both a habit and a preference. With a little perseverance and patience, you will never look back. Eventually, you will surprise yourself with new cravings for all things green!

"Genius is eternal patience."
MICHELANGELO

"Patience and perseverance have a magical effect before which difficulties disappear and obstacles vanish."
6TH US PRESIDENT, JOHN QUINCY ADAMS[9]

"You will find that your taste buds have a memory of about 3 weeks."
DR. NEAL D. BARNARD[10]

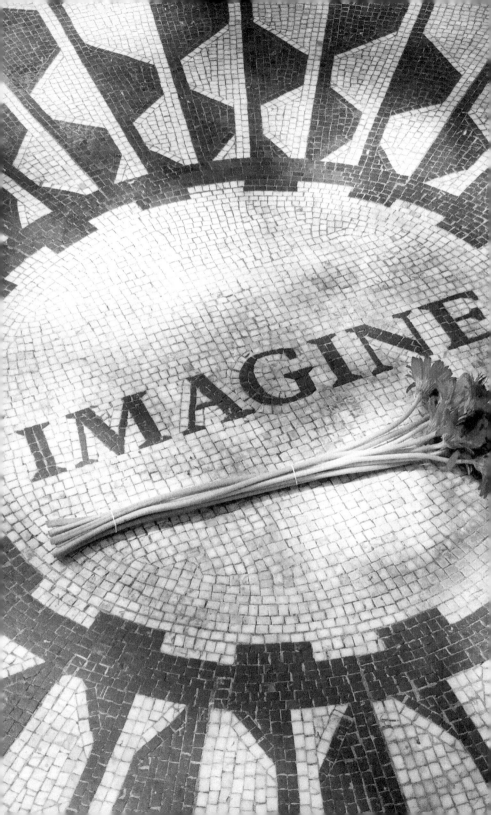

4. BELONGING:
FIND YOUR TRIBE

Connect with positive, like-minded people who can help you grow in confidence. The power of belonging should never be underestimated. To successfully transform to a cruelty-free lifestyle requires support and understanding.

No vegan is an island! Going vegan is a great opportunity to meet new friends and find support and advice along the way from fellow *REBEL VEGANS*. From Facebook groups to vegan dating apps, see this as an amazing opportunity to open up your world and create new friendships. For more detailed information, please explore our in depth Resources section at the back of this book.

If you want to go fast, go alone.
If you want to go far, go together.
AFRICAN PROVERB

"You may say I'm a dreamer, but I'm not the only one.
I hope someday you'll join us. And the world will live as one."
JOHN LENNON

"A dream you dream alone is only a dream.
A dream you dream together is reality."
JOHN LENNON

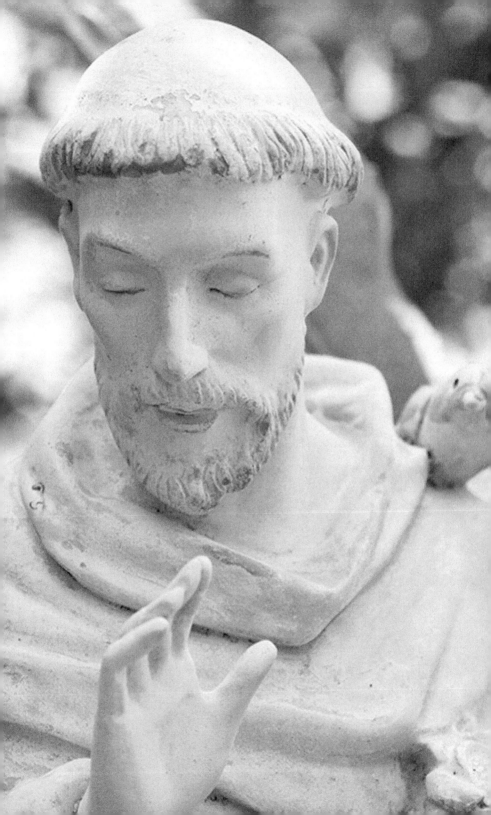

5. TEMPTATIONS:
HAVE A BACKUP PLAN

Temptations and moments of weakness happen, so make sure you have a strategy ready. My weak point is the smell of bacon. As soon as it hits me, those old habits want to take over. My strategy is to have a word with myself and remember those images in Earthlings of baby pigs being taken away from their mother. I talk myself (almost bore myself) out of any notion of indulging.

Think about the driving forces that made you decide to go vegan—this will likely be the most effective safety mechanism when temptation hits. Sometimes it helps write down your reasons for going vegan and review the list when in need. Another strategy is to have a vegan friend on speed dial for those moments of weakness.

Warning: these strategies and your commitment will be especially tested when alcohol is involved.

"Start by doing what is necessary, then what is possible, and suddenly you are doing the impossible."
ST. FRANCIS OF ASSISI[11]

"Weakness is giving in to temptation. Strength is resisting it."
GUILLERMO DEL TORO[12]

Where there is no temptation, there is no glory
ITALIAN PROVERB

Fightin

6. STAY YOUTHFUL & PRESENT:
EVERY CHILD'S WISH

If you have children, there is an extra onus and motivation to go plant-based and lead by example. A vegan diet won't just protect their health, but you'll also teach important values, such as preserving the planet and being compassionate towards other earthlings. And you'll also stay healthy and at your best for longer, which is what every child wants from their parents.

"I just decided that I was the high-risk person, and I didn't want to fool with this anymore. And I wanted to live to be a grandfather. So I decided to pick the diet that I thought would maximize my chances of long-term survival."
BILL CLINTON[13]

"The most powerful leadership tool you have is your own personal example."
JOHN WOODEN, BASKETBALL COACH AND PLAYER[14]

You will never look back on life and think, "I spent too much time with my kids."
UNKNOWN

7. ADAPT AND DEVELOP NEW SKILLS:
LEARN TO VEGANIZE

Both knowledge and charm are powerful tools. To make a lasting change, you need to feel confident in your choices and be able to respond to the skepticism and naysayers. This book's big sister, *REBEL VEGAN LIFE: A Radical Take on Veganism*, is the first deep dive into what makes vegan values so urgent in this post-pandemic world, and will prepare you for anything the skeptics throw at you.

If possible, find a vegan mentor. And, if you master the skill of veganizing, you don't need to say goodbye to your favorite restaurants or hangouts. Develop your skills to veganize with diplomacy and charm, and you will always find a tasty solution. You might even inspire your local restaurant to develop their menu, spread compassion, and inspire the next generation of *REBEL VEGANS*.

"There is no end to education. The whole of life, from the moment you are born to the moment you die, is a process of learning."
JIDDU KRISHNAMURTI[15]

"Live as if you were to die tomorrow. Learn as if you were to live forever."
MAHATMA GANDHI[16]

"I think it's a great lifestyle for long-term stability. You also have to look at everything else in your regimen, what you're putting into your body, like supplements. I'm always learning"
VENUS WILLIAMS[17]

"The Sooner You Step Away From Your Comfort Zone, The Sooner You'll Realize That It Wasn't Really All That Comfortable."
EDDIE HARRIS[18]

MAYA ANGELOU

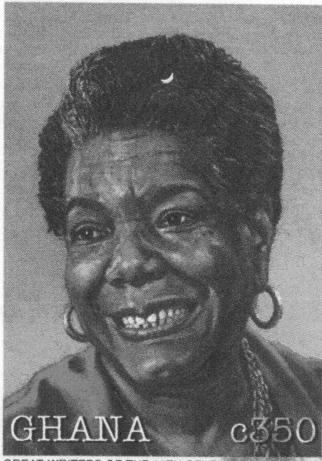

GHANA ¢350

GREAT WRITERS OF THE 20TH CENTURY

8. RECOGNIZE INSPIRATION:
CELEBRATE YOUR IMPACT

You will impact more people than you realize by going vegan. Your bold choices and courage will be an inspiration. Even the naysayers will go away and reflect on their own behavior, and need to confront their cognitive dissonance and compliance in the system. And it is one of the kindest things you can do for your loved ones, because it inspires them to become aware and improve their diet. You might even save lives.

Stand up straight and realize who you are, that you tower over your circumstances.
MAYA ANGELOU[19]

"I am a firm believer in eating a full plant-based, whole food diet that can expand your life length and make you an all-around happier person."
ARIANA GRANDE[20]

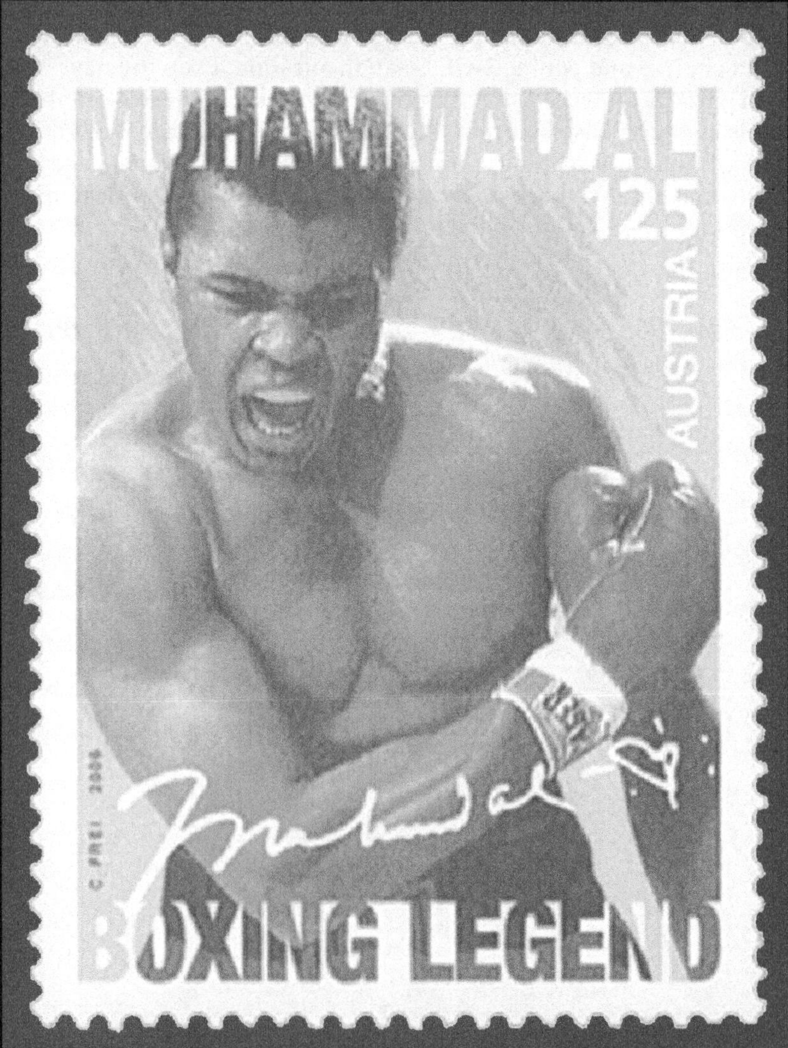

MUHAMMAD ALI
125
AUSTRIA
BOXING LEGEND

9. PAY IT FORWARD:
SUPPORT YOUR FELLOW *REBEL VEGANS*

Every vegan has unique circumstances and challenges, and has to make their own way. I believe we are stronger together, and our community should be welcoming. We share the same values, aspirations, and goals, so let's come together and celebrate each other and our movement. We are in this together, so let's make space at the table.

Service to others is the rent you pay
for your room here on Earth.
MUHAMMAD ALI

We rise by lifting others.
ROBERT INGERSOLL

There is no exercise better for the heart
than reaching down and lifting people up.
JOHN HOLMES

"Unity Is Strength... When There Is Teamwork And
Collaboration, Wonderful Things Can Be Achieved."
13-YEAR-OLD POET, MATTIE STEPANEK[21]

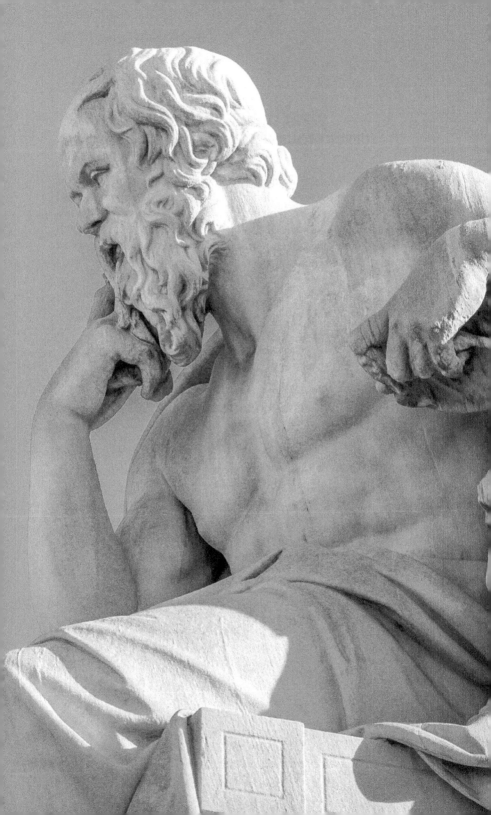

10. KNOW THYSELF:
BELIEVE IN YOURSELF AND YOUR VALUES

It takes a real sense of self to challenge the status quo or dominant way of doing things. You might need to stand up for yourself and come out as a vegan many times. The secret is to have an unshakeable belief in your ethics and reason. I recommend writing down your personal drivers and reasons for choosing this lifestyle. You can return to them time and again. Hang them on your fridge, but ultimately, you need to know—and like—yourself!

"To know thyself is the beginning of wisdom."
SOCRATES[22]

"We must be the change we wish to see."
MAHATMA GANDHI[23]

"With Every Experience, You Alone Are Painting Your Own Canvas, Thought By Thought, Choice By Choice."
OPRAH WINFREY[24]

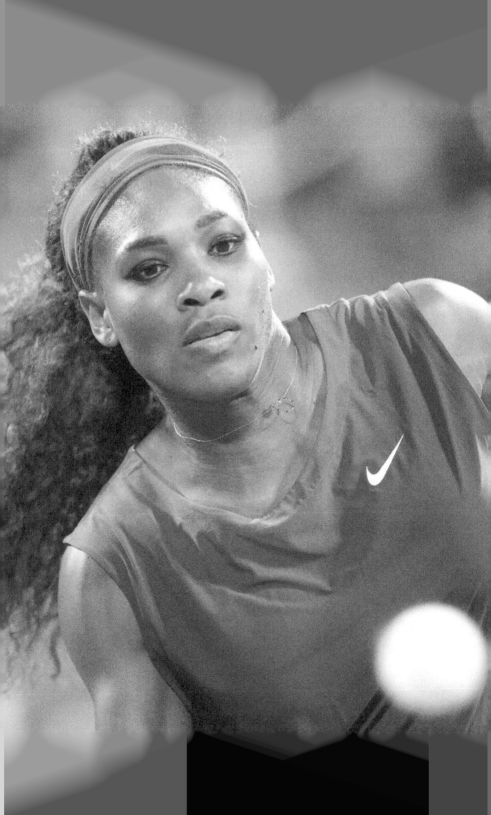

11. ULTIMATELY, GIVE IT YOUR ALL:
LIVE YOUR BEST LIFE

Whatever I do in life, I want to give it my all. It comes down to commitment and confidence in doing the right thing. Just don't forget to experiment AND have fun. Remember, like life, it's all about the journey and not the destination. Thank you for challenging and inspiring others with your brave choices.

It's pretty amazing to wake up every morning, knowing that every decision I make is to cause as little harm as possible. It's a pretty fantastic way to live.
COLLEEN PATRICK-GOUDREAU[25]

"As a new vegan, I'm enjoying exploring flavors from plants & plant-based proteins! Every journey is personal & deserves to be celebrated."
LIZZO[26]

"Once I started, I fell in love with the concept of fueling your body in the best way possible."
VENUS WILLIAMS

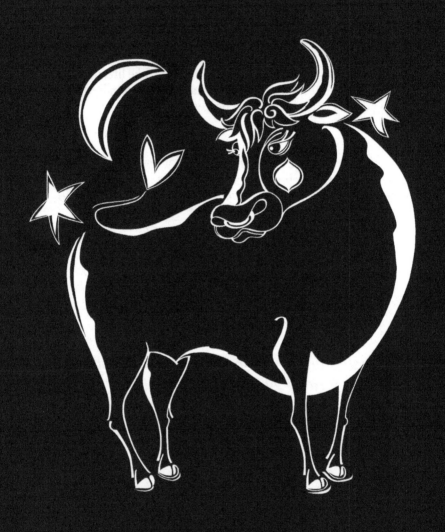

8

FINAL THOUGHTS
COMMON VALUES

"If you don't have a seat at the table, you are likely on the menu."
ELIZABETH WARREN

Our lifestyles can either protect and strengthen us or send us to an early grave. The way we produce food and the way we eat are implicated in most of the grave but preventable crises we face today. The planet's delicate ecosystems are on the brink of collapse, chronic disease is the number one killer, and viral pandemics are increasing in both frequency and severity.

Humanity is at a crossroads. We have a choice. Continue with the current status quo, or rebel, and be a force for change–on a mission to create a better world.

When Covid hit, it offered us a unique opportunity to see what is right in front of us: health is a global issue, one that is intimately connected to the health of animals and the planet. The mounting science and studies show that the best way to stop future pandemics is to stop eating animal products.[1] It is vital that we learn from Covid and make the necessary changes. This was a hard lesson, but it also points towards solutions.

Our individual health is also intimately connected to the way we eat. The standard Western diet is the biggest contributor to heart disease, cancer, obesity, diabetes, and other chronic illnesses.[2] These conditions are preventable and even reversible with a whole foods plant-based diet.[3]

Scientists have been warning for decades that our planet is suffering from the effects of our lifestyles, particularly our diet. Meat production causes deforestation, water wastage, and air pollution. Even if we stop using fossil fuels completely, we will exceed our 565-gigaton CO_2 limit by 2030, unless we drastically reduce our reliance on animal products.[4] No environmental solution will make a significant difference, unless it also includes a move away from meat production.

We must seize the small window of opportunity that we have to make real changes to the way we eat and produce food. This is our moment. We have seen through the lies: meat and dairy are not the health foods the food industry wants us to believe–quite the opposite. We can get all the nutrients we need from a well-balanced, plant-based diet. This guidebook is your springboard to a more compassionate way of eating–one that supports your health and longevity, is kind to the animals, is environmentally sustainable, and tastes amazing.

Everyone's unique journey towards veganism is like a pilgrimage home to our original, authentic selves: our compassionate and true core. I believe these are intrinsic values that we were born with, before our violent food system was normalized. Going vegan is a way to reclaim those values...and these are values that the world so desperately needs right now: compassion for ourselves and others, kindness towards all earthlings, and consideration for our planetary home.

Veganism is not just about eating more kale and avocados. It is more than just a diet. Veganism is an opportunity to see the world afresh. It is the start of a new adventure to move through our lives in a way that causes the least harm. It is a way to connect with the world ethically, compassionately, and with dignity.

You have made the bold, life-changing decision to become a *REBEL VEGAN* and invest in your health. That's a big deal, because many won't make it, or even have the opportunity to do it - you did. By being your best and most authentic self, you are a beacon of light and leading by example.

Your rebellion is a gift, both to yourself, the animals, and the planet. Your bold choice to go vegan might be the missing link for someone else to make changes or question the status quo and become another *REBEL VEGAN*. Your courageous example will challenge and inspire those around you. This is how we become a force for good and create a brave new world.

So as you start this adventure, remember to be kind to yourself, take it one day at a time, and savor every bite of your plant-based journey. I've saved you a seat at the table with all your fellow *REBEL VEGANS*.

GEORGE BERNARD SHAW
ONE OF THE ORIGINAL REBEL VEGANS!

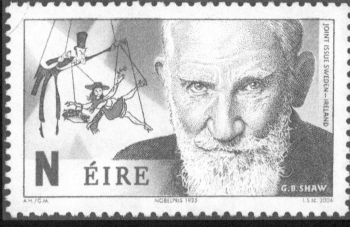

Born in Dublin in 1856, George Bernard Shaw became one of the world's greatest playwrights. He was a rebel in his own right. His plays dealt with social issues such as class privilege, inequality, education and healthcare, but his main focus was the exploitation of the vulnerable and working classes. He is the only person to be awarded both a Nobel Prize (for literature, in 1925) and an Oscar (in 1938, for his play Pygmalion, which was later turned into the film My Fair Lady).

At the age of 25, he became a strict vegetarian until his death 60 years later. He describes the vegetarian food scene in London and reports there were dozens of vegetarian restaurants, which he regularly frequented. If he were alive today, he would almost certainly identify as a vegan (the term vegan was first coined the year after he died).

He lived until the age of 94, which was almost unheard of in those days. His "extreme" diet was discussed and appraised in his obituaries around the world - probably the first time many people would have thought about this type of lifestyle.

Here are some of my favorite quotes by Shaw:[5]

A mind of the caliber of mine cannot derive its nutriment from cows.

The average age (longevity) of a meat eater is 63.
I am on the verge of 85 and still work as hard as ever.
I have lived quite long enough and am trying to die;
but I simply cannot do it.
A single beef-steak would finish me;
but I cannot bring myself to swallow it.
I am oppressed with a dread of living forever.
That is the only disadvantage of vegetarianism.

Animals are my friends... and I don't eat my friends.

You see things; you say, 'Why?'
But I dream things that never were; and I say 'Why not?'
GEORGE BERNARD SHAW, BACK TO METHUSELAH[6]

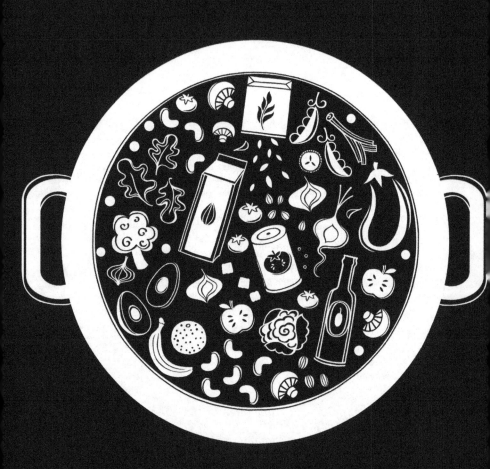

9
RECIPES

SAUCES, DIPS, SPREADS

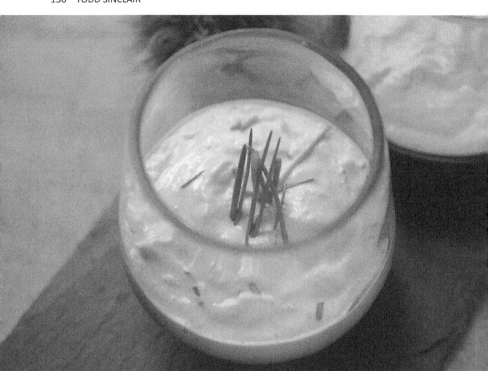

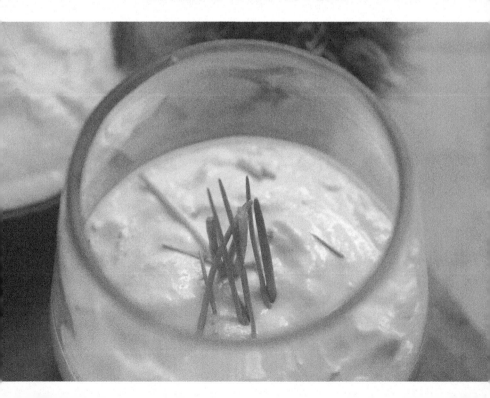

SERVES
1

Sunflower Chives Spread

Ingredients

4 tbsp chopped chives

1 small white onion

120g sunflower seeds

55ml sunflower seed oil

1 tbsp dried mixed herbs

¼ tsp nutmeg

Juice of ¼ lemon

Salt and pepper to taste

Optional: 1 clove of garlic

Directions

- In a food processor or high speed blender, add sunflower seeds, oil, and the spices.
- Pour in enough water for everything to be covered, and blend until a creamy but slightly chunky paste forms.
- Chop up the chives and add to the mix with a finely chopped onion.
- Let set for about 20 minutes before serving.

Since this spread lasts at least 5 days in the fridge, it's a great staple for sandwiches, baguettes, etc.

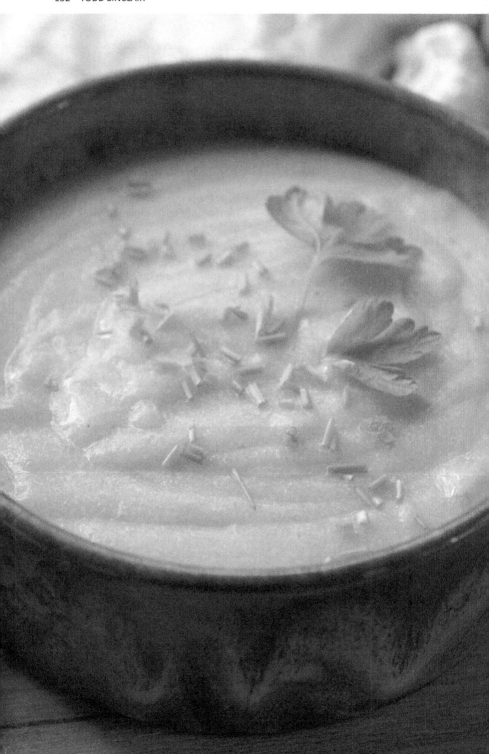

SERVES
1

Cauliflower Cheese Sauce

Ingredients

200g Cauliflower

300g Potatoes

½ medium sized white onion

¼ tsp turmeric powder

½ tsp white pepper

½ tsp Dijon mustard

1 tbsp vegetable stock

6 tbsp nutritional yeast

Pinch of sugar

Water

Salt and pepper to taste

Directions

- Peel the potatoes and add them, together with the cut cauliflower, to a medium size cooking pot.
- Roughly chop the onion, and throw it into the pot as well.
- Add enough water to cover the vegetables and add the vegetable stock.
- Cook until the potatoes and cauliflower are falling apart.
- Drain and keep save about 120 ml of the liquid.
- Add all the ingredients and spices into a blender and blend through until homogeneous.

This sauce is especially great for burgers, vegan mac and cheese, nacho platters, or in tacos!

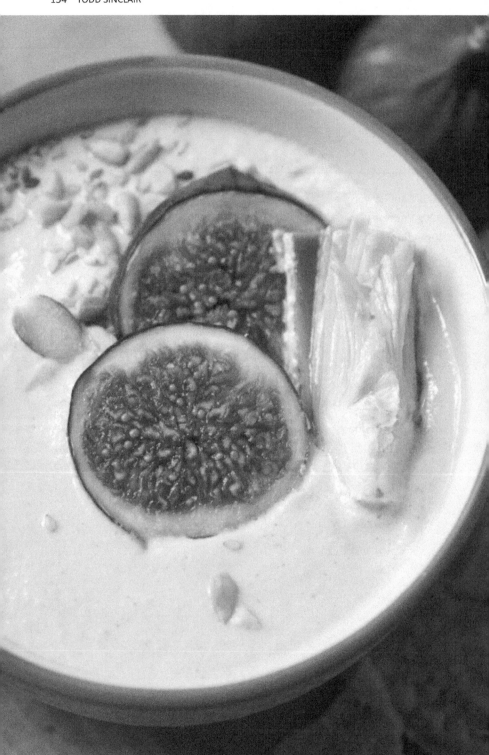

Artichoke Dip

SERVES
1

Ingredients

125g Cashews

75g Firm Tofu

90g Artichokes from a jar

**~200ml Plant milk of choice
(I recommend oat or soy) –
unsweetened**

2 tbsp Nutritional yeast

**½ tsp of each garlic and onion
powder**

**1 ½ tbsp sweet paprika
powder**

**2-3 tbsp sunflower seed or
olive oil**

Optional: Chili flakes

Directions

- Soak the cashews in hot water (ensuring all the cashews are fully covered) for at least 1.5 hours.
- Rinse and drain them, and bring all the ingredients together in a high-speed blender.
- Blend until nice and smooth, and season with salt and pepper to taste.
- This is a great recipe to use for get-togethers, parties, or spontaneous picnics!
- Simply serve them with some vegan nachos or crackers on the side.
- And it also goes really well on bagels, sandwiches, or baguettes.

We love it combined with some fresh figs, dried tomatoes, and nuts.

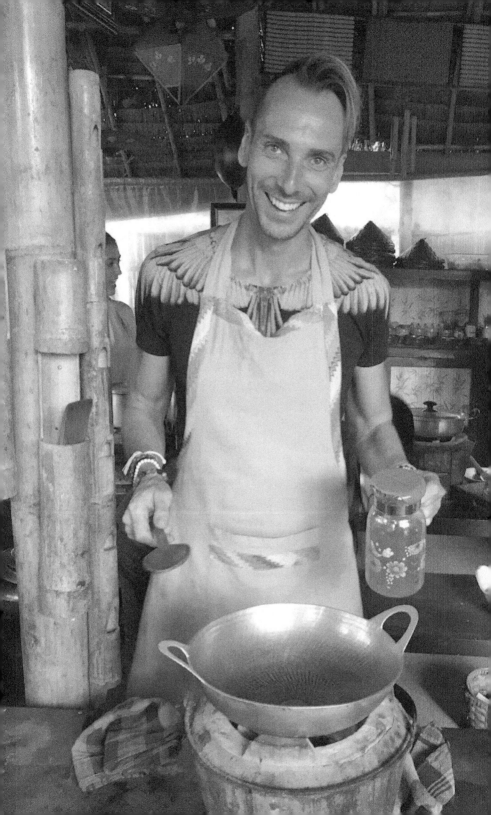

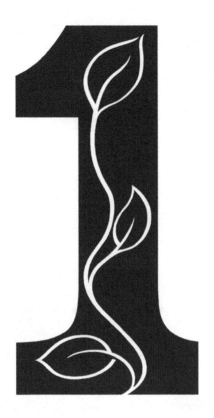

WEEK 1
CUT OUT EGGS AND DAIRY AND
START OFF WITH A VEGAN BREAKFAST

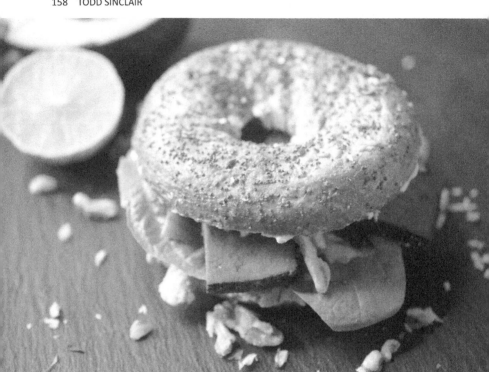

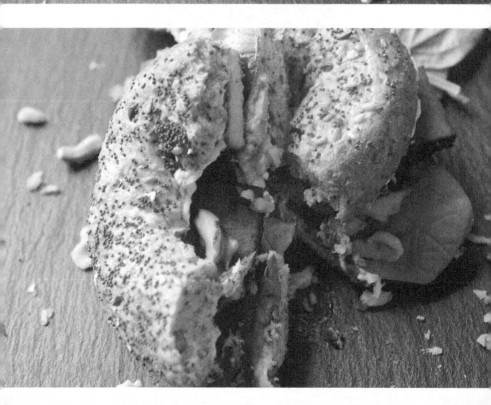

SERVES
1

Avocado Bagels with marinated tofu thins

Ingredients

Vegan bagel of choice

70g Smoked Tofu

½ Avocado

Fresh greens of choice (e.g. baby leaf spinach)

2-3 Walnuts

Juice of ¼ lime

Few slices of a small red onion

For the marinade:

1 tsp soy sauce

½ tbsp Worcester sauce

1 tsp nutritional yeast

½ tsp of each garlic and onion powder

½ tsp smoked paprika powder

1 tbsp sunflower seed oil

Directions

- Cut the tofu into equal sized slices that fit onto your bagel of choice.
- Prepare the marinade by mixing all the ingredients together, and let the tofu slices soak in it for at least 30 minutes.
- In the meantime, cut your bagel in half and toast until crispy golden brown.
- Mash the avocado together with lime juice and a pinch of salt.
- Grill the marinated tofu from both sides over medium heat and start assembling your bagel by starting with the artichoke cream, followed by greens, mashed avocado, tofu, onions, and walnuts. Enjoy!

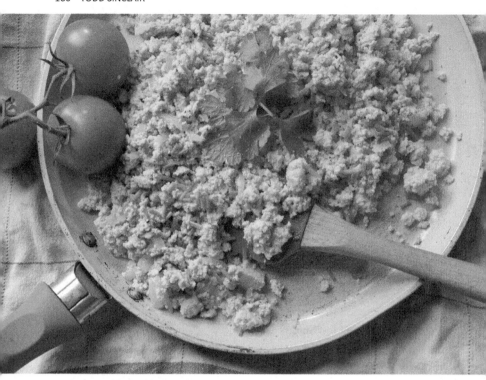

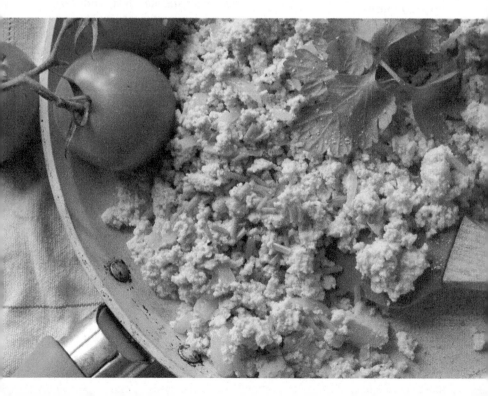

Tofu Scramble

**SERVES
1 - 2**

Ingredients

½ white onion

1 block firm tofu

3 tbsp nutritional yeast

1 tbsp sunflower seed oil or a slice of vegan butter

A pinch of each turmeric and garlic powder

Salt and pepper to taste

Directions

- Cut the onion in rounds and slice in half.

- Add some oil to a pan and throw in the onion together with 1 block mashed (scrambled) firm tofu.

- Add all the spices and stir until homogeneous.

- Let the covered scramble cook for about 5 minutes over low-medium heat, mixing through every now and then.

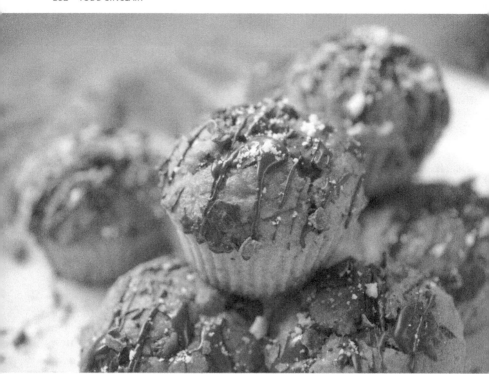

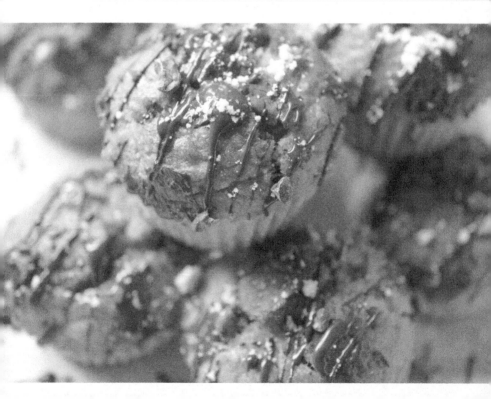

**SERVES
1**

GF Banana Choco Muffins

Ingredients

165g oats or oat flour

200 ml plant milk (unsweetened)

1 tsp lemon or lime juice

1 ½ tsp baking powder

1 tsp baking soda

80g cane sugar

50-60g nut butter (e.g. almond)

½ tsp cinnamon powder

2 tbsp sunflower seed oil

2 small – medium size bananas (very ripened)

50g of dark chocolate (e.g. 70%)

Directions

- Preheat your oven to about 180*C.
- Mix the milk together with lemon juice and set aside.
- If you're using oats for this recipe, make sure to first ground them into a flour.
- Mix the oat (flour) together with the rest of the dry ingredients, then add in the mashed bananas and milk.
- Chop up your chocolate and stir it into the batter.
- Grab your muffin tin or molds and fill them up before transferring them into the oven to bake for at least 30 to 40 minutes.

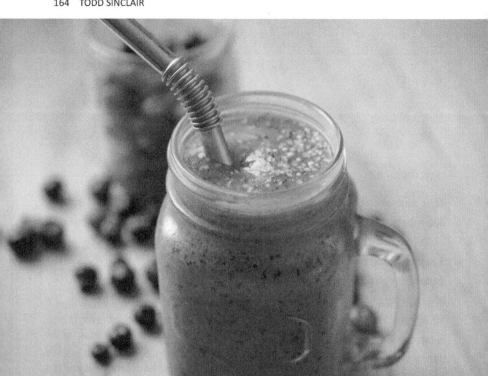

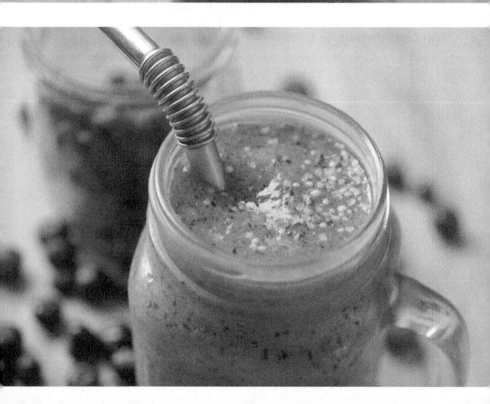

**SERVES
1**

Berry Smoothie

Ingredients

1 large frozen banana

120g frozen mixed berries (or any other red berry)

220 ml almond milk

¼ tsp cinnamon

Optional: hemp seeds

Directions

- Blend everything together in a high-speed blender and drink right away.

Smoothies are such a great "dish" as you can bring them with you wherever you go (as long as you keep them in an insulated jug/bottle)!

They're also a great way to add more greens or antioxidants into your diet!

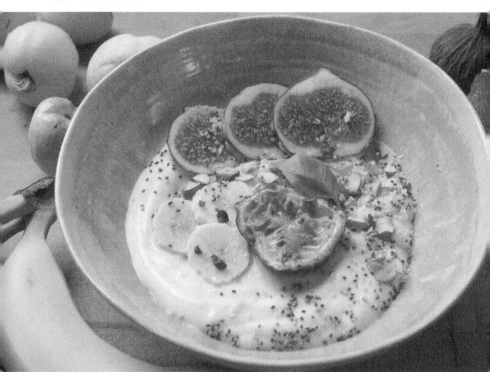

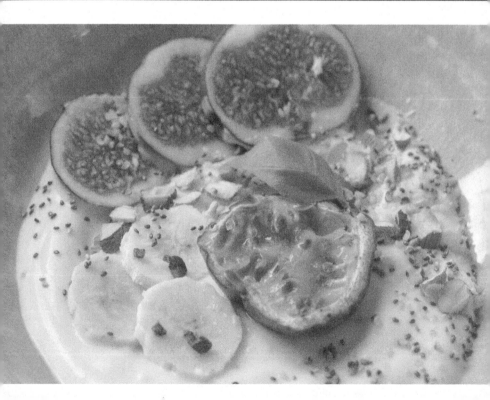

Yoghurt Bowl

**SERVES
1**

Ingredients

180g coconut yogurt

½ banana

Fruit of choice, e.g. figs, passionfruit

2 tbsp crushed or shaved nuts

1 tsp of each hemp and chia seeds

Optional: dark chocolate nibs

Directions

- Add the yogurt to a serving bowl, chop up your favorite fruits, and add some nuts and seeds for healthy fats!

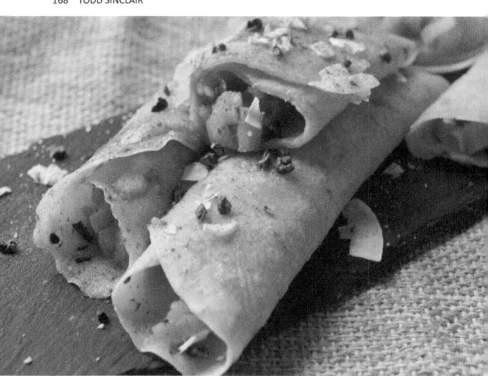

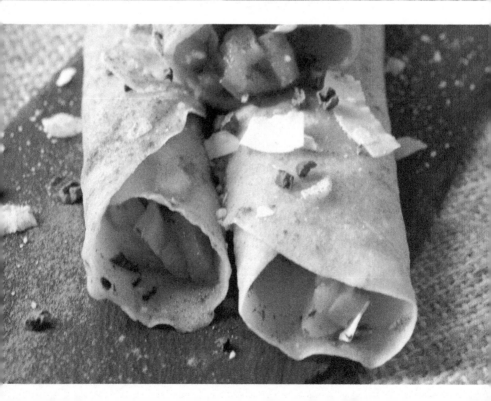

**SERVES
2 - 4**

Crepes with cooked apples

Ingredients

200g spelt flour

300 ml plant milk

2 tbsp cane or coconut blossom sugar

Pinch of salt

2 small apples

1 tsp coconut oil

Few raisins

1 tbsp cane or coconut blossom sugar

Pinch of each nutmeg and cinnamon

Directions

- Prepare the crepes batter by simply adding all the dry ingredients into a mixing bowl before pouring in the milk.

- Whisk together and cook in a lightly greased pan over low-medium heat on both sides.

- Chop up the apples and transfer them into a small pot together with the raisins, cinnamon, nutmeg, coconut oil, and sugar.

- Cook down over low-medium heat and keep covered until you have finished the crepes batter.

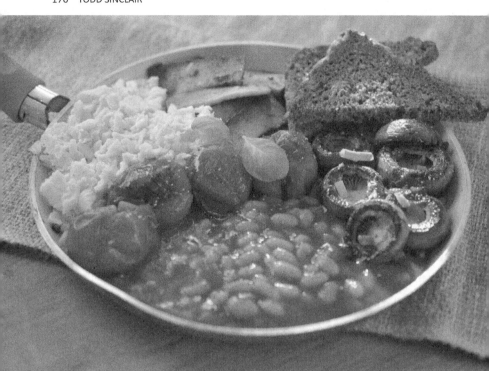

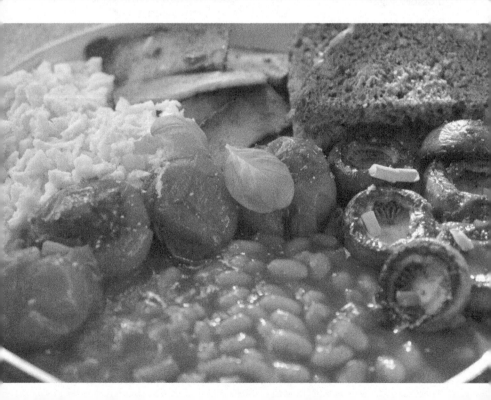

**SERVES
1-2**

Veganized English Breakfast

Ingredients

175g brown button mushrooms

Medium thick slice of vegan butter

Tofu scramble

Marinated smoked tofu

4 small tomatoes

150g white beans in tomato sauce

Directions

- Cook mushrooms and tomatoes in a little bit of vegan butter for extra flavor!
- Then simply check out the recipes for the tofu scramble and for the smoked marinated tofu.
- You only have to prepare the marinade we have used for the tempeh medallions, cut your smoked tofu into slices and grill on both sides until crispy.
- Heat up the beans and assemble with some fresh bread on the side, and optionally, some freshly cut chives.
- Enjoy!

Not only is this a classic, it's also really healthy. It provides fiber, iron, proteins, and healthy carbs. It will keep you satiated for a long time!

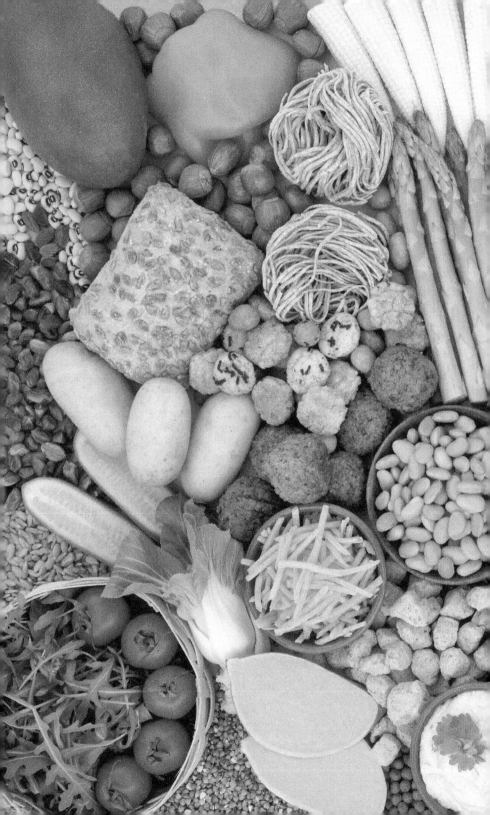

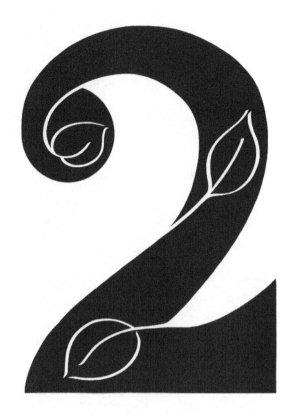

WEEK 2
CUT OUT RED MEAT AND
IMPLEMENT PLANT-BASED LUNCHES

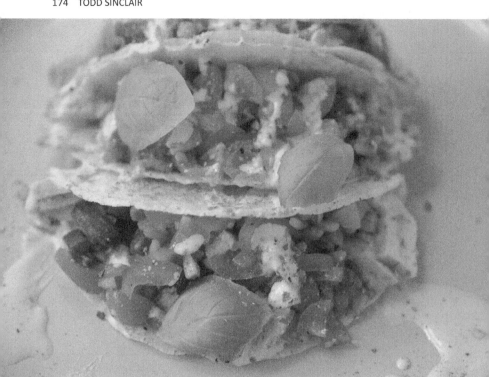

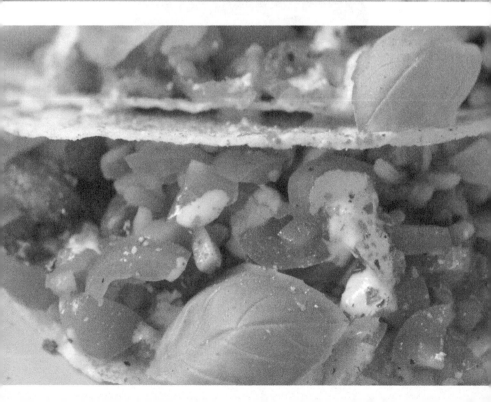

SERVES 2

Hard-shelled Tacos with Avocado and Salsa

Ingredients

1 bell pepper

1.5 small red onion

2 cloves of garlic

100g tinned kidney beans

2 tsp tomato paste

1 tsp caraway

2 tsp smoked paprika

1.5 tbsp Worcester sauce

Olive oil

6-8 brown button mushrooms

1 Avocado

8 cherry tomatoes

Juice of ¼ - ½ lime

Salt and Pepper to taste

Fresh basil or coriander

Directions

- Chop bell pepper, 1 clove of garlic, and onion into small cubes.
- Cook together with some olive oil in a medium size cooking pan over medium heat.
- Cover with a lid and let simmer until the peppers start to soften.
- Add in tomato paste, spices (except salt*), Worcester sauce, and mushrooms.
- Mix well and stir in kidney beans once the mushrooms are almost cooked.
- Turn off heat and keep covered with a lid while preparing your salsa!

For the Salsa

- Start by chopping the tomatoes into small cubes.
- Do so with the other garlic clove and half of another red onion too.
- Mix it all together with some olive oil, salt and pepper, and fresh greens, such as coriander or basil.
- You can add some fresh chilies here for a bit of heat!
- Assemble as you please and enjoy together!

The artichoke dip is a great combination with this, as it's not too dominant in flavor, yet adds some creaminess.

The marinade of the tempeh medallions works great as a sauce for tacos and nachos too!

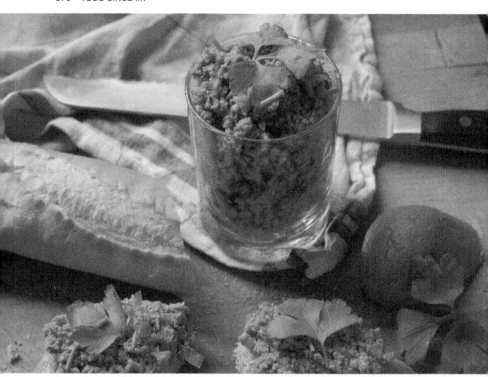

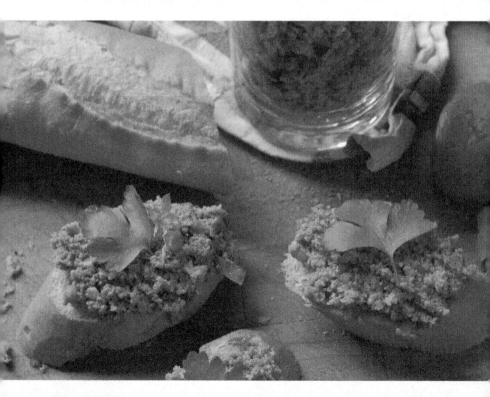

**SERVES
1**

Hearty Walnut Paste
on baguette

Ingredients

75g Walnuts

120g smoked tofu

½ red onion

1 tbsp soy sauce

1,5 tbsp tomato paste

1 tsp liquid smoke

½ tbsp smoked paprika powder

¼ tsp cumin

Pinch of garlic powder

2 tbsp sunflower seed oil

Fresh parsley to serve with

Directions

- Add everything to a high speed food processor and blitz through
- (use the "pulse" setting here if your food processor has one).
- Make sure the texture remains chunky, but sticks together when pressed between your fingers.
- Store in fridge to keep fresh!

Serve it on the side of some fresh bread! We love a good French baguette or a rustic, crunchy dark bread with it.

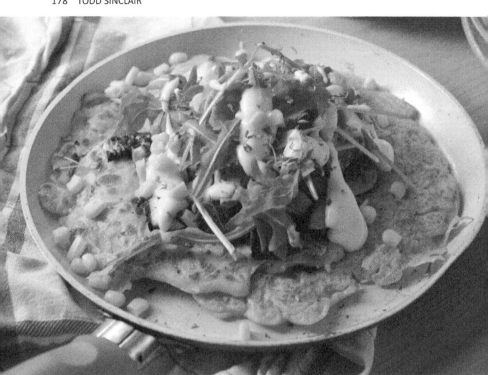

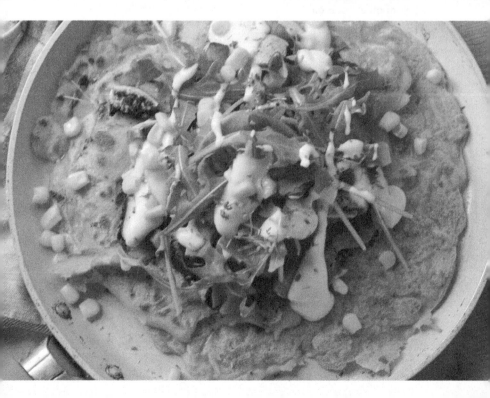

**SERVES
2**

Sweet Potato – Basil Pancakes

Ingredients

80g shredded or shaved sweet potato

100g spelt flour

1 tbsp nutritional yeast

1 tbsp sunflower seed oil

½ tsp each garlic and onion powder

Pinch of nutmeg and turmeric

175 ml nut milk unsweetened (e.g. oat)

Few leaves fresh basil

6 medium size mushrooms

Handful fresh greens, e.g. arugula

100g soy yogurt

1 garlic clove

Squeeze of ½ lemon

Salt and pepper to taste

Directions

- Mix the soy yogurt together with 1 clove of freshly minced garlic and lemon juice.
- Set aside.
- In a large mixing bowl, mix flour, spices, and plant milk.
- Add in the shredded sweet potato and whisk well.
- Add some oil to a pan over medium heat and bake the pancakes from both sides.
- Serve with fresh greens and your garlic infused lemon yogurt!

This is a great Sunday morning / brunch dish!

It's hearty, fresh, and takes seconds to prepare.

Feel free to change up the toppings: marinated vegetables, sautéed spinach with mushrooms, etc.

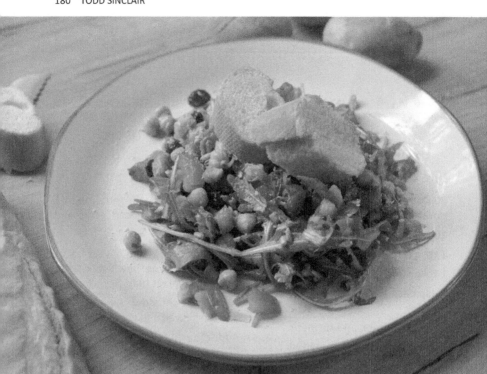

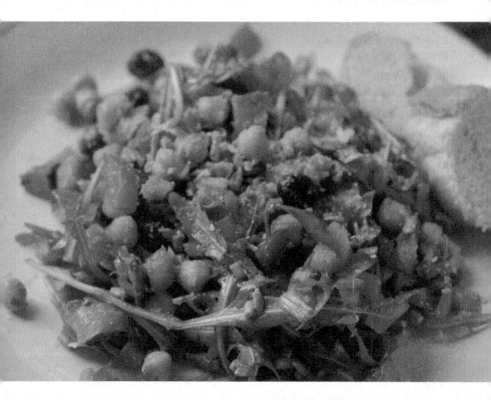

SERVES 2

Arugula Chickpea Salad

Ingredients

3-4 handful fresh arugula

10 cherry tomatoes

175g precooked chickpeas

Kalamata olives

25g dried cranberries

2 tbsp sunflower or pumpkin seeds

2 tbsp olive oil

2-3 tbsp balsamic vinegar

Salt and pepper to taste

Directions

- Wash and dry the arugula and transfer into a medium size mixing bowl.
- Chop tomatoes into quarters and olives in half – add to the salad.
- Throw in the rest of the ingredients and simply adjust with salt and pepper!

You can use this recipe as a main for a warmer day, or as a side salad to a soup as well!

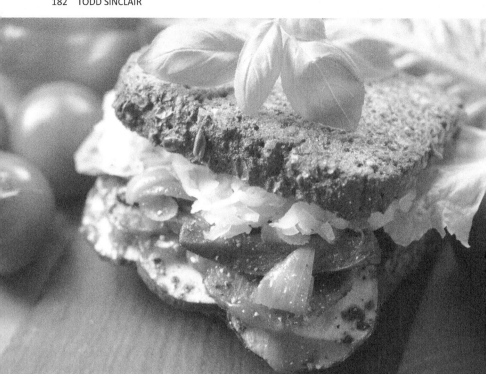

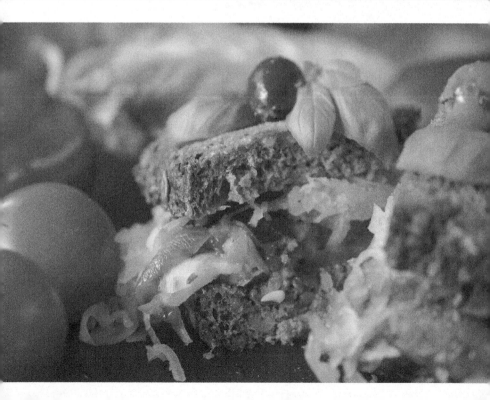

**SERVES
1**

Sandwich with marinated Tofu

Ingredients

2 slices bread of choice

4 sundried tomatoes

75g firm tofu

2 leafs Roma salad

1 tomato

Grilled vegetables of choice (e.g. eggplant, bell pepper)

Cucumber

1 tsp Dijon mustard

2 tsp balsamic vinegar

1 tbsp liquid smoke

1 ½ tbsp maple syrup

½ tsp of each garlic and onion powder

Salt and pepper to taste

Directions

- To marinate the tofu, mix all the liquids and spices in a mixing bowl, and let the tofu soak in it for at least 1 hour (you can also prepare this the night before and store it in the fridge).

- Cut your vegetables into Juliennes and grill them in a pan with a touch of oil.

- In the meantime, toast your bread and chop up the tomato and cucumber into rounds.

- Grill the tofu from both sides and assemble your sandwich together with the rest of the ingredients!

Such a good dish to take to work / school with you or to enjoy together on a picnic!

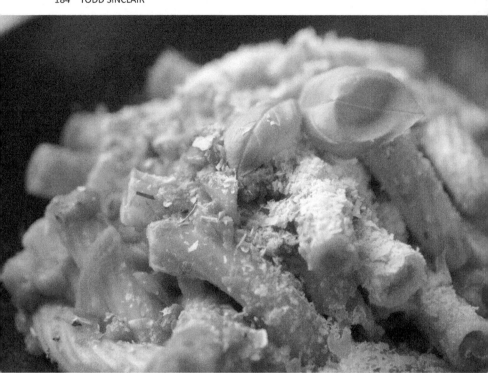

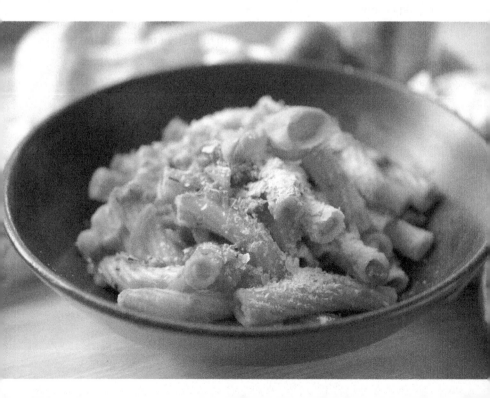

**SERVES
2**

Lentil Pasta
in tomato sauce

Ingredients

2 servings of pasta (of choice)

**250-300g passata italiana /
tomato sauce**

1 tbsp tomato paste

2 garlic cloves

1 medium size white onion

**150g cooked red or brown
lentils**

1 tsp dried Italian herbs

Salt and pepper to taste

2-4 tbsp pasta water

Directions

- Cook two servings of pasta according to the directions on the package.

- To prepare the sauce, simply sauté the chopped up garlic and onion in a little bit of olive oil over medium heat.

- Once translucent add in tomato paste, herbs and mixed cracked pepper.

- Stir in the passata, followed by lentils.

- Pour a little bit of the pasta water into the sauce, then strain the pasta just a little before they're fully cooked (so they don't get too soft when being mixed with the sauce).

- Serve with some fresh herbs and nutritional yeast on top!

Pasta dishes are great to take to work or school as they can be enjoyed cold as well, don't take up too much space and can easily be reheated another time.

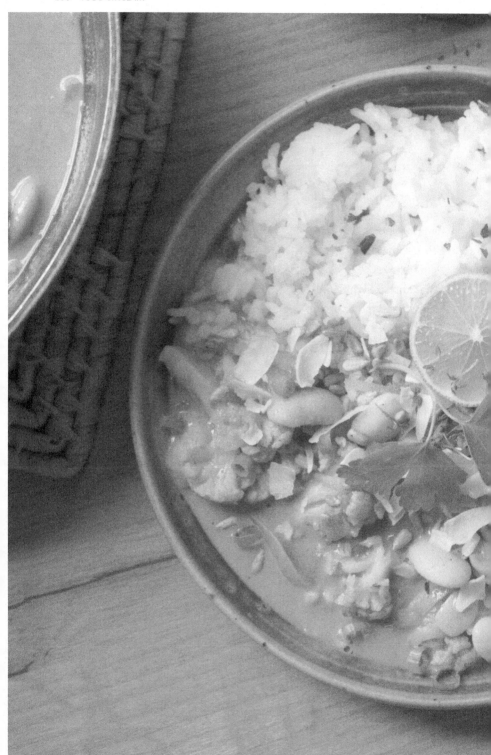

Cauliflower
White Bean Curry

**SERVES
2 - 3**

Ingredients

1 tin white beans

450g cauliflower

1 large white onion

2 cloves garlic

1 tbsp caraway

½ tsp nutmeg

1 tbsp smoked paprika

3 tsp yellow curry powder

2 tsp cane sugar

1,5 tbsp vegetable stock

150 ml water

Fresh ginger

Fresh coriander

Directions

- Chop up onion and garlic and add to a large cooking pot with the oil and spices.

- Stir together and throw in the chopped up cauliflower.

- Pour in about 150ml of water together with the vegetable stock, and let it all cook down until the cauliflower starts to soften.

- Whisk in some thinly sliced ginger and the pre-cooked beans, and let sit for about 25 minutes without heat.

- Keep the pot covered and serve with rice and fresh lime on the side.

A lovely family dish that can be prepared in bigger batches in advance, so that you can simply freeze or store the rest in the refrigerator for another time!

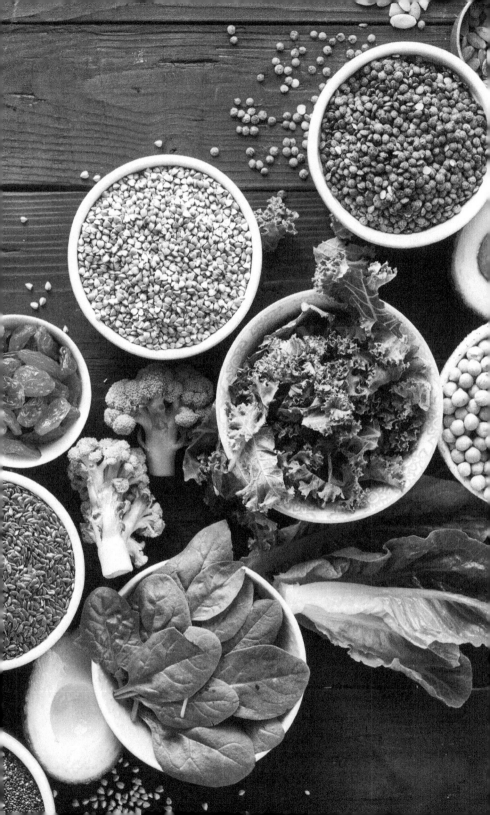

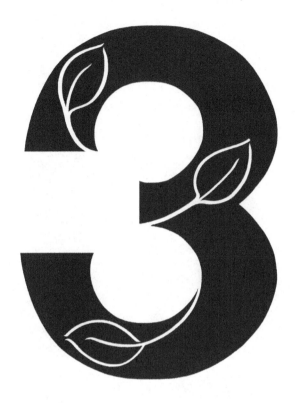

WEEK 3
CUT OUT ALL LAND ANIMALS AND GO FOR VEGAN DINNERS AND SUPPERS

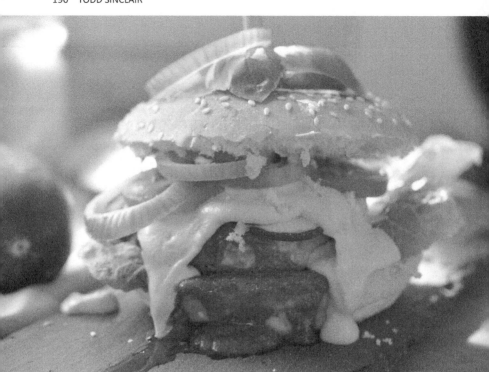

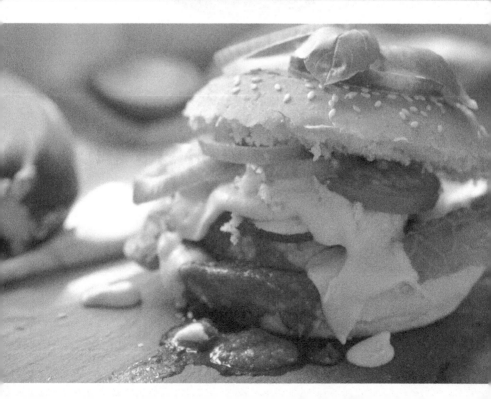

**SERVES
4**

Rebel Vegan Burgers

Ingredients

Vegan Burger Buns

Tomatoes

Roma Salad

1 Red Onion

400g Firm Tofu

Optional: pickled cucumbers

For the marinade:

2 tbsp Tomato paste

2 tbsp Liquid smoke

1 tbsp Sunflower seed oil

1 tbsp Worcester sauce

1 tbsp Nutritional Yeast

1 tsp   White Pepper

½ tsp of each onion and garlic powder

Salt and Pepper to taste

Directions

- Prepare the marinade by mixing all the ingredients together in a small mixing bowl (should be big enough for you to soak the tofu in).

- Note: You might want to use a little water if your marinade is getting too thick.

- Cut four equal sized rounds out of your blocks of tofu.

- Pat them dry and let them soak in the marinade for at least 1 hour. Flip and cover with marinade from both sides from time to time.

- Grill them in a pan from both sides over medium heat and keep it covered with a lid.

- Assemble your burgers as you please – done!

The Cauliflower – Cheese Sauce goes really well with this recipe!

Simply reheat the sauce over low-medium heat until warm enough, and drizzle over the patties while layering the ingredients.

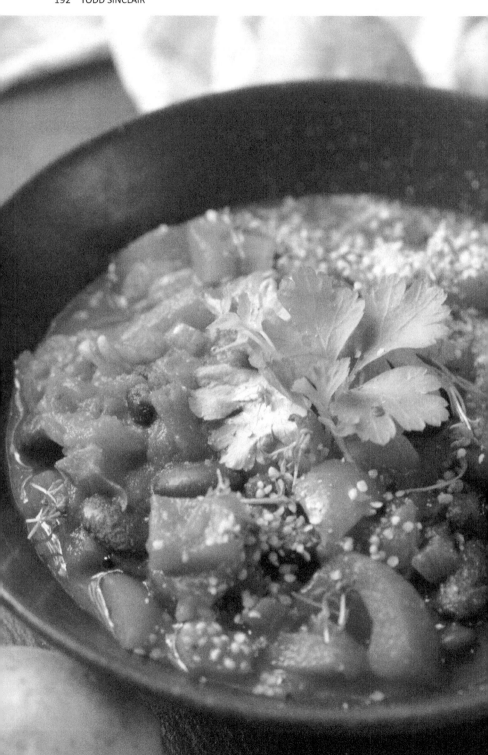

SERVES 2 - 4

Chili Sin Carne

Ingredients

1 Red Pepper

275g cooked kidney beans

1 large white onion

2 cloves of garlic

2-3 Tbsp Tomato Puree

250g tinned chopped tomatoes

2 Tbsp Vegetable stock

100-150 ml Water

1-2 Tbsp Olive Oil

1,5 Tbsp Smoked Paprika Powder

1 Tsp Miso Paste

1 Tsp caraway

Pinch of Sugar

1 Bay Leaf

Salt and Pepper to taste

Directions

- Chop the onion into medium sized pieces and mince the garlic.
- Throw both together in a large cooking pot with some olive oil and sauté until translucent.
- Cut your pepper into bite size cubes and add to the pot with all the spices (including vegetable stock), miso, and tomato paste.
- Mix well, add the tinned tomatoes and water, and stir in the bay leaf.
- Cover with a lid and cook for about 10 to 15 minutes, or until the peppers start to feel a little soft.
- At this point, mix in your pre-cooked kidney beans so they heat up together with the rest.
- Turn off the heat and let everything sit for another 20 minutes (with the lid on).
- Serve with some fresh greens, such as coriander and parsley!

This is a really great party dish too, and I'm sure no one will taste the difference to a traditional chili con carne!

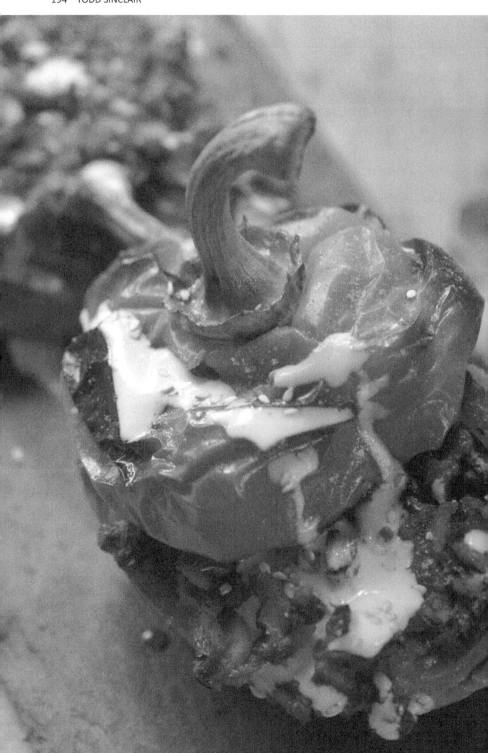

Stuffed Peppers

**SERVES
2 - 3**

Ingredients

150g pre-cooked lentils

2 large bell peppers

1 serving rice (listed on the package)

1 medium sized carrot

1 medium sized white onion

2 cloves of garlic

1 – 2 tbsp olive oil

3 tbsp vegetable stock

2 tsp liquid smoke

1 tbsp smoked paprika powder

½ tsp caraway

1 tbsp tomato paste

Salt and pepper to taste

Juice of ½ lime

Water

Directions

- Start by pre-heating your oven to about 200C.
- Cut open the peppers to remove their seeds, and glaze with a bit of oil. Sprinkle some salt before transferring them into the oven to grill while preparing the filling.

Filling

- Slice the onion into rings, then cut in half.
- Chop the carrot into small cubes and mince the garlic.
- Add everything to a large cooking pan with some olive oil, and let simmer over low-medium heat with a lid on until onion and garlic start to lose color.
- Mix in your pre-cooked lentils together with all the spices, tomato paste, liquid smoke, and cooked rice.
- Whisk everything together, adjust with salt and pepper as you please, and turn off the heat.
- Add in the lime juice, then take the peppers out to stuff them.
- Transfer back into the oven for about 30 to 40 minutes.

Our Cauliflower-Cheese sauce goes really well with this recipe too!

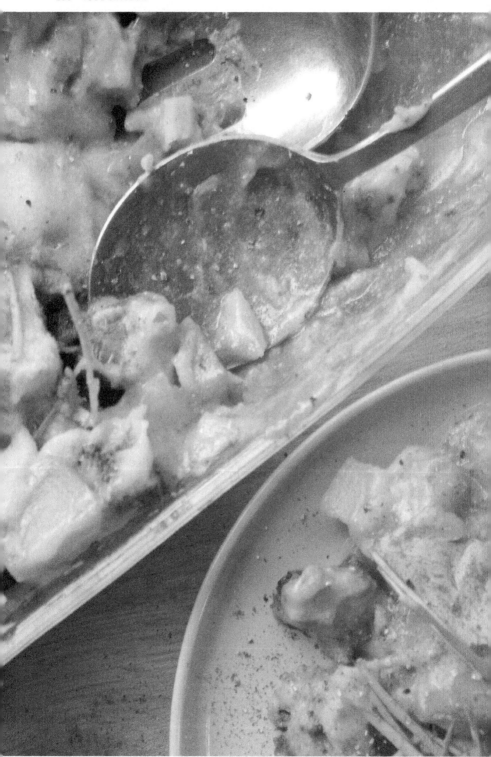

**SERVES
4**

Broccoli Zucchini Loaf
with cheese sauce

Ingredients

300g potatoes

300g broccoli

2 cloves of garlic

1 medium sized zucchini

1 medium sized white onion

1 tbsp smoked paprika powder

½ tbsp white pepper

2 tbsp olive oil

~ 100 ml plant milk unsweetened

Salt and pepper to taste

Directions

- Preheat your oven to 185*C.

- Chop potatoes, broccoli, and zucchini into small cubes, making sure the potato pieces are a little smaller than the rest, as they take the longest to cook.

- Finely slice your garlic, chop up the onion and mix it all together in a large mixing bowl, together with the spices and oil.

-

- Add a little bit of plant milk to a casserole dish and transfer your vegetables into the oven for about 30 minutes – stir around every once in a while.

- After 30 minutes, pull out from the oven and pour the cheese sauce over.

- Let cook for another 20 minutes – done!

I recommend serving this with fresh greens, e.g. some flat leaf parsley or baby leaf spinach. It will add a nice crunch to it!

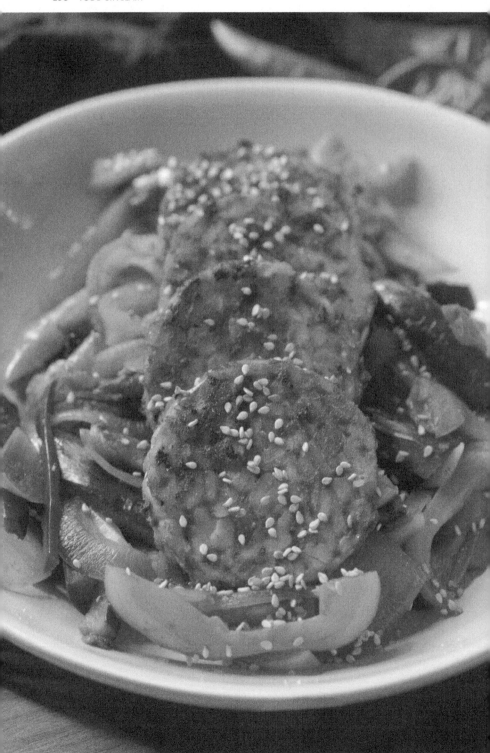

**SERVES
1 - 2**

Tempeh Medallions
on grilled Vegetables

Ingredients

200g tempeh

2 tbsp tomato paste

1 tbsp liquid smoke

2 tbsp Worcester sauce

1 tbsp plant oil (e.g. sunflower seed)

½ tsp Dijon mustard

2 tsp smoked paprika powder

1 tsp maple syrup

Optional: 1 tsp cayenne pepper

Water to dilute

½ large eggplant

2 peppers, e.g. red and yellow

1 medium size of both red and white onion

Salt and pepper to taste

Optional: freshly minced garlic

Directions

- Mix all the listed ingredients together in a bowl, chop the tempeh into slices or rounds (depending on what shape it comes in) and marinade from both sides for at least 1h.

- Make sure you flip them every once in a while, so both sides are evenly covered and soaked.

- In the meantime, prepare your grilled vegetables by simply cutting them into Julienne strips and add them into a pan with a touch of oil.

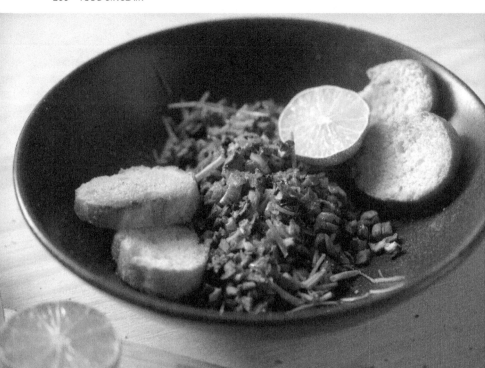

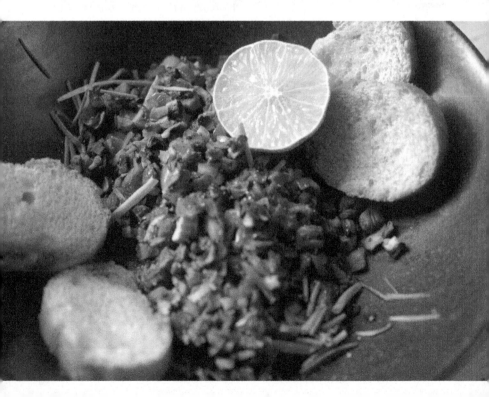

**SERVES
2**

Mushroom Tartar

Ingredients

**650g / 23 oz brown button
mushrooms**

3 shallots

2,5 tbsp sunflower seed oil

1 tsp lemon juice

**1 tbsp freshly chopped
parsley**

1 – 2 tbsp freshly chopped

Salt and pepper to taste

Directions

- Clean and gently wash the mushrooms, then chop into small cubes.

- Add some oil to a pan and grill the mushrooms until all liquids have evaporated.

- In the meantime, dice your shallots and add them to the pan just before the mushrooms are done.

- Finely chop up the fresh greens and bring all the ingredients together in a mixing bowl before seasoning with salt and pepper.

- Drizzle in some lemon juice and let sit for about 5 minutes before serving.

This dish goes great together with some fresh baguette and margarine!

It's also great for parties or as a starter!

.

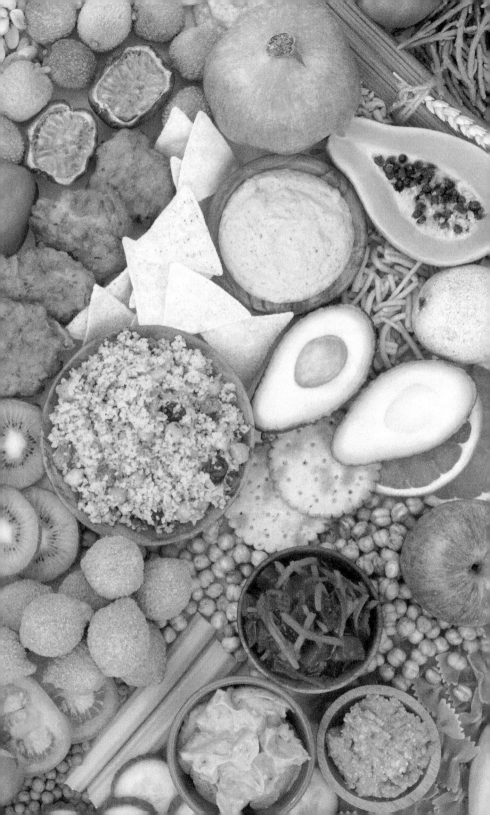

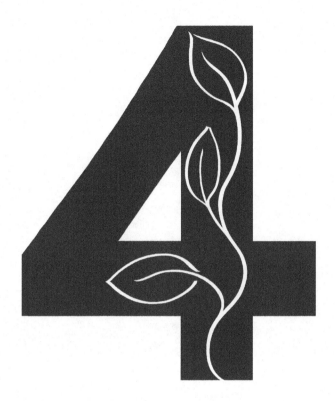

WEEK 4
CELEBRATION DINNER!

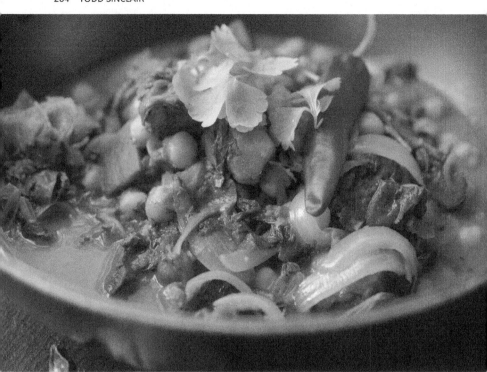

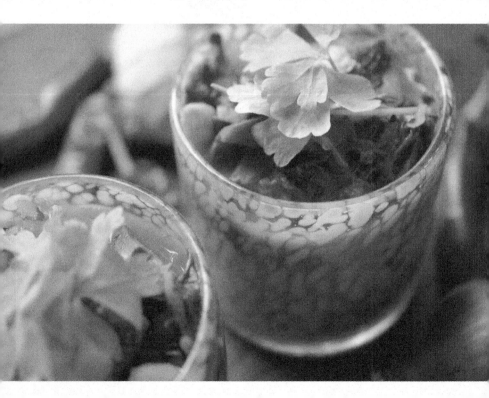

Todd's Curry

**SERVES
3 - 4**

Ingredients

2 tbsp coconut oil

2 tins chickpeas

1 tin jackfruit

250g baby leaf spinach

½ tin coconut milk

½ tin chopped tomatoes

2 medium size white onions

2 medium size tomatoes

2 cloves of garlic

2 tbsp mustard seeds

2 tbsp cumin

1 tbsp garam masala

1 tbsp curry powder

1 tbsp turmeric

1 tsp freshly chopped ginger

Optional: 2 green chilies

Directions

- In a large cooking pot, mix the coconut oil, chopped onions, minced garlic, and all the spices.
- Stir and cook until caramelized.
- Add in the ½ tin chopped tomatoes, freshly chopped tomatoes, and ginger.
- Let everything cook down over medium heat with a lid on.
- Stir every once in a while, then pour in ½ tin of coconut milk, 1 tin of each blended and unblended chickpeas and the jackfruit.
- Mix together and add the spinach afterwards.
- Cover with a lid, reduce the heat to low and let simmer for another 10 minutes.

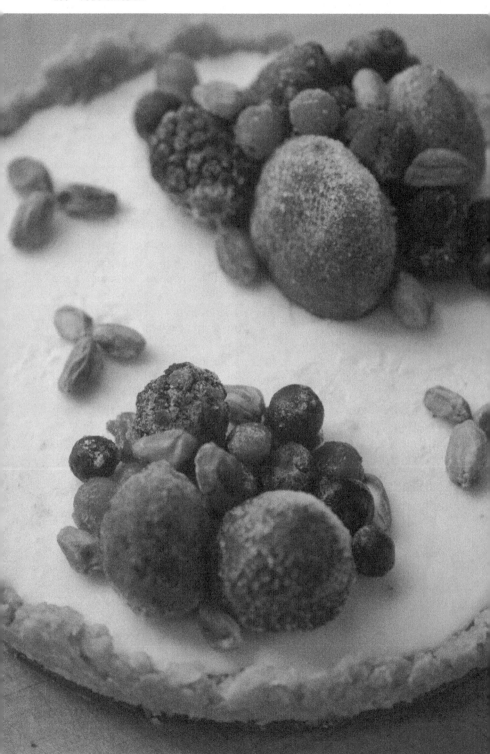

**SERVES
1**

Raw Vegan Coconut Berries Cake

Ingredients

90g Cashews
2 tbsp Maple syrup
3 tbsp coconut yogurt
2 tbsp coconut oil
1 tsp vanilla extract
½ tsp rose water
Juice of ½ lemon

Base

150g shredded oats
130g pitted dates
½ tsp cinnamon
Pinch of salt
1 ½ tbsp coconut oil

+ Frozen berries of choice

Directions

- Soak the cashews in hot water for at least 1.5 hours.

- To prepare the base, mix all the ingredients (base) in a food processor until the mixture starts sticking together when pressed in between fingers.

- Press into a small ring baking tin with removable bottom and freeze for about 40 minutes.

- In the meantime, prepare the filling by draining the cashews and adding them to a blender with all the other ingredients.

- Pour onto the base and freeze for another 1,5h before decorating.

- Once you decorated the cake, freeze for another 40 to 60 minutes or until the filling is stiff enough.

Make sure to defrost the cake at room temperature for at least 10 minutes before cutting it so it doesn't break.

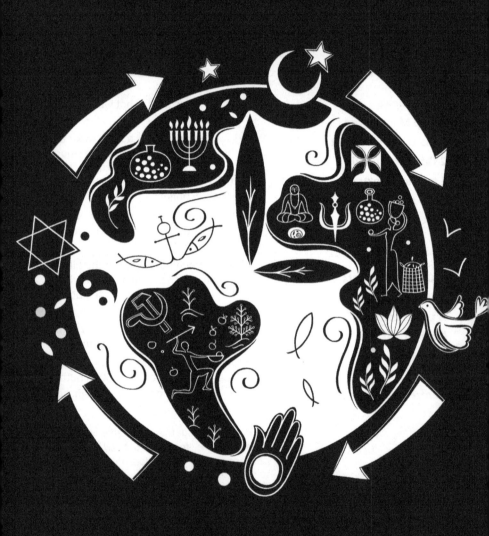

10

RESOURCES

In my years of veganism and travel, I have collected a treasure trove of resources to help me along my way. I've done my best to share this knowledge and information with you in my Rebel Vegan series. To help you quickly access this information while on the go, I have compiled all of the resources mentioned in this guide into one compact resource section. Feel free to dogear these pages and references when needed in your life and adventures.

WEBSITES

Save these websites to your Favorites Bar before preparing your next vegan vacation. These resources will make the planning process considerably easier.

- **Plant Based Health Online**: The top plant-based doctors in the UK offering healthcare and lifestyle advice to overcome chronic illnesses and certain cancers. *PlantBasedHealthOnline. com*

- **Plant Based Healthcare Professionals**: This patient/ public resources are incredible with factsheets, news roundups and webinars etc on healthy plant-based diets. *PlantBasedHealthProfessionals.com/factsheets*

- **Vegan Fitness**: This is a UK based community with discusses everything vegan and fitness related. Their forums cover all aspects of a vegan lifestyle with an emphasis on sports training, health, and fitness. You can answer all your questions here! *www.veganfitness.net/*

- **HappyCow**: This website is helpful for finding vegan restaurants around the world. It is user-sourced, so you can add or update restaurants, as well as read customer reviews. Bonus, this website comes in app form too. *HappyCow.net*

- **VegVisits**: The Airbnb for vegans. Book unique homestays and accommodations with locals in over 80 countries. *VegVisits.com*

- **Vegan Meetups, Couchsurfing, and Traveling**: A Facebook community with 7,000 members. Vegan gatherings and open Couchsurfing opportunities are listed here. Members also discuss travel experiences and questions. You have to request membership for this group. *facebook.com/groups/974772789309783*

- **Barnivore**: A searchable directory of wines, beers, and liquors denoting which are vegan-friendly. *barnivore.com*

- **Vegan Travel Facebook Group**: The group currently has over 35,000 members. The content discusses all things vegan related, and many members are more than happy to answer your questions. *facebook.com/groups/vegantravel*

- **Vegan Travel**: Virtual vegan community with reviews, blog posts, videos, and more for planning your vegan trips. *VeganTravel.com*

- **Foundation for Intentional Community**: Want to live with other vegans? Interested in growing your own food? How about popping in for a weekend visit? Use this website to access a global directory of intentional communities. The advanced search option lets users narrow the search to vegetarian and/or vegan communities. *ic.org*

- **Food Labels Exposed**: Use this website put together by A Greener World to help you navigate the confusing world of food labels. *aGreenerWorld.org/wp-content/uploads/2015/03/AGW-Food-Labels-Exposed-2017-EMAIL-SCREEN-8-31-2017.pdf*

- **Animal Welfare's Consumer's Guide**: The Animal Welfare Institute has put together a listing of all food labels and what they mean, explaining which are legal terms and which are made up by the food companies. *awiOnline.org/content/consumers-guide-food-labels-and-animal-welfare*

- **Vegan Calculator**: Ever wished you could measure the impact you've made in your vegan or vegetarian journey? Now you can. Measure your impact at: *VeganCalculator.com*

- **Book Different**: This website rates hotels in terms of their eco-friendliness. *BookDifferent.com*

APPS

Download these apps on your phone ASAP! These resources will help you with just about everything - booking a hotel room, scoring a yummy vegan meal, communicating in a foreign language, and more.

- **Vegan Passport**: This is a digital food card available in various languages to help you explain your dietary preferences. The passport explains in detail which ingredients vegans do and don't eat in 78 different languages.

- **Google Translate**: You can speak or type words and phrases to be translated into over 100 languages. You can even point your camera at a block of text and have it translated for you in real-time. Be sure to download the language pack for the specific language you need, so that the app can be used offline as well.

- **AirVegan**: Use this app when heading to the airport. AirVegan shows how vegan-friendly an airport is. It lists all places that offer vegan options, and even tells you where they are located. Some of you may have encountered this app back when they only supported airports in the United States. Good news - the app went international with its listings back in 2018.

- **Food Monster**: This app provides the user with a database containing over 8,000 vegan recipes. While it isn't travel-related, it can aid you in your travels by providing quick and budget-friendly meals when you select the filters 'Less Than Five Ingredients' or 'Quick Meals'.

- **VeganXpress**: This app only works for travel in the US. It lists all vegan menu choices at 150 chain restaurants throughout the US. The database goes into great detail about all the possible vegan options. It also includes a food guide for supermarkets, and another guide for various alcoholic drinks.

- **V-Cards**: Vegan Abroad: V-cards, vegan cards in this case, are translation cards to help you order food abroad. This is a similar concept to the food cards offered up in the Hot Spots chapter of this guide, only they offer translations in over 100 languages on demand.

- **Veganagogo**: This is another translation app - because you can never have too many. Users choose from a list of pre-written questions and statements, making it easier to use than Google Translate in some scenarios.

- **Foodsaurus**: Standing in the grocery aisle at a foreign market completely unsure of what the ingredient list on the pre-made boxed meal lists? Whip out your phone and scan the ingredient list with Foodsaurus, and the app will translate the label to your language of choice.

- **Veggly**: Can't imagine dating an omnivore? Looking for a romantic partner that can hold you accountable in your vegan journey? Check out Veggly, a vegan dating app currently available in 181 countries.

- **Vegan Check**: This app double checks that products are entirely vegan before purchasing. It also includes services such as tattoo studios and salons.

- **Vegan Pocket**: Vegan Pocket scans barcodes to check if the product is vegan. No more reading confusing food labels! Just scan, and done.

- **abillion | Impact made easy**: This app lets you search for vegan brands and products near you, wherever you are around the world. After finding a vegan product on the app, you can even read customer reviews.

VOLUNTEERING

Want to get involved? Use these websites to find volunteer opportunities in the vegan community.

- **WWOOF**: Worldwide opportunities to volunteer on organic farms. Typically, room and board are offered in exchange. You must create an account for each country you would like to search for hosts in, and a subscription fee is required. *wwoof. net*

- **WorkAway**: Worldwide opportunities to volunteer at organic and non-organic farms, homesteads, communities, non-profit organizations, and more. Room and board are typically offered in exchange. Sometimes hosts offer an hourly wage in addition to this. A small subscription fee is required. *WorkAway.info*

- **HelpX**: HelpX is the same concept as WorkAway (above), without the opportunity for an hourly wage. Room and board are usually offered, and a small subscription fee is required. *helpx.net*

- **Voluntouring**: This blog keeps an up-to-date listing of organizations looking for volunteers. The listing has a tab for listings that strictly adhere to vegan principles. *voluntouring.org*

- **International Volunteering**: Facebook group listing international vegan-based volunteer opportunities. *facebook.com/groups/217244375670902*

- **Grassroots Volunteering**: Database of international grassroots volunteer experiences. Search the site for vegan-centered opportunities, or contact hosts to see if vegans can be accommodated. *GrassRootsVolunteering.org*

- **WorldPackers**: Volunteer experiences and programs for travelers in over 100 countries. *WorldPackers.com*

VEGAN TOURS

These vegan tour guides and agencies take the work and planning out of your adventure, leaving nothing but fun and delicious plant-based food for you. Each has detailed websites listing all of their services and destinations! Even if you don't plan on booking with an agency, they are worth looking at for inspiration and ideas.

P.S. These are tour groups offering international opportunities. If you already have a destination in mind, do a quick Google search for vegan tour guides there. I bet you'll find even more resources!

- **Vegan Food Tours**: European Vegan City Tours. *VeganFoodTours.com*
- **Vegan Adventure Tours**: Specialising in epic tours through Latin American and UK micro tours. *VeganAdventureHolidays.com*
- **Intrepid Travel**: International tour company does several vegan tours annually. *IntrepidTravel.com/vegan-food-adventures*
- **The Nomadic Vegan**: Website for Vegan Tours, Vegan Cruise, and Vegan-friendly tour operators. *TheNomadicVegan.com/vegan-tours*

FESTS AND EVENTS

A great way to have fun and immerse in the vegan culture while traveling is to attend a festival or event. Below I list a number of resources for finding events in several destinations. This list is not exhaustive! Reference it, and then do further research to find even more fun items to add to your travel calendar.

- **Vegan Festivals Directory:** *vegan.com/blog/festivals*
- **VegEvents International:** *VegEvents.com*
- **International Listing:** *vegan.com/blog/festivals*
- **Vegan Society International Listings:** *VeganSociety.com/ whats-new/events*
- **HappyCow International Listings:** *HappyCow.net/events*
- **UK Vegan Events:** *VeganEventsUK.co.uk*
- **USA Vegan Events:** *AmericanVegan.org/vegfests*
- **Australia Vegan Events:** *VeganAustralia.org.au/events*

FILMS:

- Cowspiracy (Netflix)
- Seaspiracy (Netflix)
- Earthlings (Free stream on http://www.nationearth.com/)
- The Game Changers (Netflix)
- What The Health (YouTube)
- Forks Over Knives (YouTube)
- The End of Meat (YouTube)
- Meat Me Halfway (YouTube/ Amazon Prime)
- Eating Our Way to Extinction (Amazon Prime)
- The Invisible Vegan (Amazon Prime)
- The Animal People (Amazon Prime)
- A Prayer for Compassion (Amazon Prime)
- My Octopus Teacher (Netflix)
- Okja (Netflix)

My Top Pic: Babe / Babe: Pig in the City (Amazon or Netflix)

BOOKS

CLASSIC READS:

- **Vegetable Diet: As Sanctioned by Medical Men, and by Experience in All Ages (1838) by William A Alcott**: The world's first book to advocate a vegetarian diet! It's been reprinted by The American Antiquarian Cookbook Collection and still in print today.

- **Diet for a Small Planet (1971) by Frances Moore Lappe**: A groundbreaking book arguing that world hunger is caused by the meat industry. It was the first time that meat was shown to be unhealthy and leading to global poverty.

- **Animal Liberation (1975) by Peter Singer**: This book is widely considered the founding philosophical statement of its ideas within the animal liberation movement. Singer claimed that industrial farming is responsible for more pain and misery than all the wars of history put together.

- **Main Street Vegan: Everything You Need to Know to Eat Healthfully and Live Compassionately in the Real World (2012) by Victoria Moran**: Holistic health practitioner Victoria Moran offers a complete guide to making this dietary and lifestyle shift with an emphasis on practical "baby steps," proving that you don't have to have a personal chef or lifestyle coach on speed dial to experience the physical and spiritual benefits of being a vegan.

- **The China study: The Most Comprehensive Study of Nutrition Ever Conducted and the Startling Implications for Diet, Weight Loss and Long-Term Health (2004) by T. Colin Cambell**: This novel takes the reader through a twenty-year study which looked at mortality rates from cancer and other chronic diseases from 1973 to 1975 in 65 counties in China. The China Study examines the link between the consumption of animal products (including dairy) and chronic illnesses such as coronary heart disease, diabetes, breast cancer, prostate cancer, and bowel cancer.

MODERN READS:

- **Why We Love Dogs, Eat Pigs, and Wear Cows by Melanie Joy**: The social psychologist who coined the word and hidden belief system of "carnism." (Her YouTube channel is good as well).

- **Beyond Beliefs: A Guide to Improving Relationships and Communication for Vegans, Vegetarians, and Meat Eaters by Melanie Joy, PhD**: This book is recommended for anyone living with or in close relationships with non-vegans.

- **We Are the Weather: Saving the Planet Begins at Breakfast by Jonathon Safran Foer**: This book explains how collective human action is the only way to save the planet, and as the title suggests, this begins with what is on our plates.

- **Eating Animals by Jonathon Safran Foer**: Part memoir, part investigative report. This book is a moral examination of vegetarianism, farming, and the food we eat.

- **Sex Robots & Vegan Meat: Adventures at the Frontier of Birth, Food, Sex, and Death by Jenny Kleeman**: This novel is an investigation into the forces driving innovation in the core areas of human experience.

- **Some We Love, Some We Eat, Some We Hate: Why It's So Hard to Think Straight About Animals by Hal Herzog**: A scientist in the field of anthrozoology offers a controversial exploration of the psychology behind the ways we think, feel, and behave towards animals.

***ALL RESTAURANTS, APPLICATIONS, WEBSITES, AND OTHER RESOURCES ARE UP TO DATE AS OF THE TIME OF PUBLISHING.

TIMES ARE TURBULENT, AND THEREFORE DYNAMIC. ALWAYS DOUBLE CHECK TO ENSURE ORGANIZATIONS ARE STILL IN OPERATION.

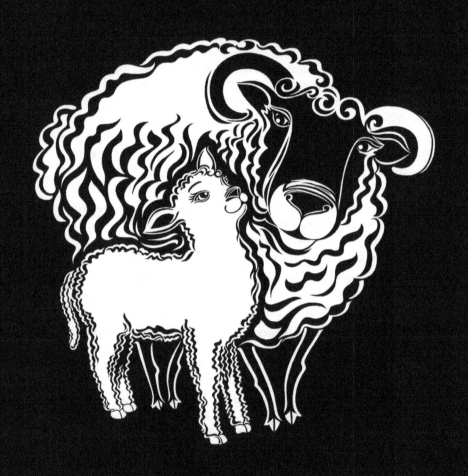

11

APPENDICES

APPENDIX 1: HANDY FOOD LISTS

ESSENTIAL AMINO ACIDS AND PLANT SOURCES[1]

ESSENTIAL AMINO ACID	PLANT FOOD SOURCES
Isoleucine	Tofu, lupin beans, lentils, oats, oat bran, buckwheat, lima beans, chickpeas, Swiss chard, whole wheat, pistachios, spinach, wild rice, quinoa, sunflower seeds.
Leucine	Tofu, oats, navy beans, adzuki beans, white beans, buckwheat, lentils, mung beans, broad beans, teff grain, kamut grain, pumpkin seeds, hemp seeds.
Lysine	Tofu, edamame beans (soy beans), green peas, lupin beans, navy beans, adzuki beans, lentils, lentil sprouts, white beans, split peas, buckwheat, oats, black beans, mung beans, quinoa, hemp seeds.
Tryptophan	Tofu, oats, buckwheat, pumpkin seeds, sea vegetables, whole wheat, walnuts, lentils, mung beans, chickpeas, sesame seeds, chia seeds, sunflower seeds, quinoa, potatoes, pine nuts, cacao.
Valine	Tofu, oats, buckwheat, navy beans, lupin beans, white beans, oat bran, adzuki beans, lentils, lentil sprouts, kidney beans, lima beans, black beans, peanuts, flax seeds, brown rice, spinach, cashew nuts.
Threonine	Tofu, lupin beans, oats, buckwheat, white beans, navy beans, lentils, adzuki beans, split peas, corn, chickpeas, soy sprouts, black eyed peas, broad beans, teff grain, hemp seeds, wheatgerm, pumpkin seeds, peanuts.
Histidine	Tofu, oats, buckwheat, lentils, white beans, kidney beans, adzuki beans, mung beans, pea sprouts, wild rice, chia seeds, almonds, sunflower seeds, whole wheat, peanuts.
Phenylalanine	Tofu, edamame beans (soy beans), oats, navy beans, lupin beans, white beans, kidney beans, pinto beans, buckwheat, lentils, lentil sprouts, mung beans, cornmeal, hemp seeds, peanuts, quinoa, millet, sunflower seeds, almonds.
Methionine	Tofu, oats, oat bran, brazil nuts, teff grain, wheatgerm, corn, buckwheat, hemp seeds, white beans, kidney beans, sesame seeds, lentils, green peas, sweet potatoes, millet.

ESSENTIAL MACRO-NUTRIENTS AND PLANT SOURCES

PLANT PROTEIN	COMPLEX CARBOHYDRATES	HEALTHY FATS
Lentils (brown, red, yellow, green) Chickpeas Black beans Black-eye beans Kidney beans Cannellini beans Butter beans Navy beans Split peas Snap peas Green beans Lima beans Pinto beans White beans Broad beans Mung beans Adzuki beans Peanuts Hemp seeds Chia seeds Quinoa* Buckwheat* Amaranth* Soy / tofu / tempeh Pasta and noodles made from beans or lentils	Root vegetables (sweet potatoes, carrots, celeriac, parsnips, beetroot, turnips, potatoes, yam, pumpkin, squash) Whole grains (amaranth*, barley, buckwheat*, rice, bulgur wheat, corn, polenta, kamut, millet, oats, quinoa*, rye, sorghum, spelt, teff, triticale, couscous) Pasta and noodles made from whole grains (wheat, spelt, wheat), as well as brown rice and buckwheat Sourdough bread or organic bread made from whole grains Oat crackers Fruits (especially ones with edible seeds like berries, apples, watermelon, papaya, kiwi)	Olive oil Coconut oil Avocado oil Walnut oil Sesame oil Flaxseed oil Almonds Hazelnuts Brazil nuts Cashew nuts Pecan nuts Macadamia nuts Pine nuts Pistachios Peanuts Pumpkin seeds Sunflower seeds Hemp seeds Chia seeds Sesame seeds Coconut (fresh, dried, or coconut milk) Avocado Omega-3: Seaweed and algae (sea salad, kombu, wakame, nori, spirulina) Chia seeds Hemp seeds Walnuts Flax seeds

* Amaranth, buckwheat, and quinoa are pseudo-grains - they are used like grains in cooking, but are actually seeds. This is why they are excellent sources of both protein and complex carbohydrates.

ESSENTIAL MICRONUTRIENTS AND PLANT SOURCES[2]

MICRONUTRIENT	WHAT IT DOES	BEST SOURCES
Vitamin A	• Supports eyes and prevents age-related macular degeneration. • Helps the body make antibodies that neutralize or fight pathogens. • Needed to produce new red blood cells.	Sweet potatoes, carrots, spinach, kale, squash, Swiss chard, collard greens, squash, romaine lettuce, cantaloupe melon, bell peppers, parsley, broccoli, papaya, pink grapefruit, chives, apricots, tangerine, peaches, sour cherries, plantain
Vitamin B1 (thiamin)	• Helps your body convert fat, sugars, and protein from food into usable energy. • Has a role in brain cells' structure and function.	Sunflower seeds, sesame seeds, peanuts, black beans, peas, lentils, cabbage, navy beans, kidney beans, tofu, flaxseed, sweet potato, Brussels sprouts, yeast extract, spirulina, parsley, rice, oat bran, cornmeal, oats, barley, kamut
Vitamin B2 (riboflavin)	• Like all B vitamins, it helps the body convert food into useable energy. • Helps recycle glutathione (the body's own powerful antioxidant). • Helps prevent anemia.	Spinach, beetroot greens, mushrooms, sweet peppers, radish, yeast extract, parsley, chives, lychees, corn, wheat bran, soybeans, tempeh, almonds, sesame seeds, yeast extract (such as Marmite), spirulina
Vitamin B3 (niacin)	• Essential for energy production. • Protects against free radicals.	Mushrooms, green peas, potatoes, corn, asparagus, sweet potato, hot chili peppers, tomatoes, peanuts, brown rice, sunflower seeds, sesame seeds, wheat bran, buckwheat, spelt, wild rice, yeast extract
Vitamin B5 (pantothenic acid)	• Important for energy production, particularly from fats. • Helps make anti-stress hormones and vitamin D. • Maintains healthy skin and hair.	Shiitake mushrooms, portobello mushrooms, onions, avocado, sweet potato, potatoes, broccoli, cauliflower, papaya, squash, tomatoes, endive, dried apricots, lentils, peas, rye, rice, oat bran, wheat bran, amaranth, buckwheat, spelt, wheat, teff, sunflower seeds, sesame seeds, spirulina

Vitamin B6 (pyridoxine)	• Helps the body to produce red blood cells. • Breaks down carbohydrates for energy. • Required for the production of key neurotransmitters. • Helps the liver eliminate toxins.	Cabbage, bok choi, sweet potato, potatoes, spinach, cauliflower, bell peppers, broccoli, squash, bananas, chives, shallots, prunes, apricots, garlic, pistachios, sunflower seeds, sesame seeds, wheat bran, rice, yellow corn, amaranth, buckwheat, yeast extract
Vitamin B12 (cobalamin)	• Keeps the cardiovascular system healthy by helping blood carry oxygen to all your cells. • Prevents homocysteine build up (an inflammatory marker linked with cardiovascular disease). • Essential for DNA production. • Keeps brain cells and nervous system healthy.	Small amounts found in some mushrooms and fermented foods (kimchi, sauerkraut, miso, kombucha) - however a good quality B12 supplement is recommended.
Folic Acid (Folate)	• Supports healthy brain and nervous system function. • Reduces homocysteine levels and protects the cardiovascular system. • Essential for fetus development during pregnancy. • Helps form red blood cells.	Asparagus, spinach, leeks, edamame beans, radish, sweet peppers, parsley, avocado, black beans, kidney beans, wheat germ, enriched wheat flours, corn, rice, quinoa, wild rice, millet, lentils, pinto beans, chickpeas, yeast extract, agar agar seaweed, sunflower seeds, sesame seeds, hazelnuts, chestnuts
Vitamin C	• Powerful antioxidant - protects the body against free radicals. • Needed for collagen production and skin health. • Required to make serotonin (our mood neurotransmitter). • Supports a strong immune system and helps to fight infections.	Papaya, bell peppers, broccoli, strawberries, pineapple, oranges, kiwis, melon, cauliflower, parsley, kale, celery, Brussels sprouts, chives, mustard greens, red cabbage, lychees, red currants, lemons, grapefruit, peaches, papaya, strawberries, pineapple, apples, clementines, chestnuts, thyme, dill

Vitamin D	• Helps the body absorb calcium to keep bones and teeth strong. • Involved in blood sugar control (deficiency may be a factor in diabetes). • Helps white blood cells mature and function.	Shiitake mushrooms, fortified breakfast cereals, plant milks, plant yogurts, and enriched flours - however, a good quality vegan Vitamin D supplement is recommended.
Vitamin E	• Potent antioxidant - protects cell membranes against free radical oxidation. • Reduces levels of bad cholesterol (LDL). • Keeps skin supple.	Spinach, chard, avocado, peanuts, turnip greens, asparagus, sweet peppers, broccoli, fresh coriander, apricots, olives, brown rice, quinoa, rye, oat bran, whole grain wheat, agar agar seaweed, sunflower seeds, almonds, hazelnuts
Vitamin K	• Needed for normal blood clotting. • Helps keep bones strong.	Kale, spinach, collard greens, chard, parsley, broccoli, Brussels sprouts, radicchio, chicory greens, prunes, rhubarb, avocado, pears, pine nuts, pumpkin seeds, cashew nuts, soy beans, miso, natto (fermented soy), split peas, kidney beans, buckwheat, rye
Calcium	• Supports bone and teeth health. • Critical for acid-alkaline balance of the body. • Regulates nerve signals.	Collard greens, spinach, chives, radishes, leeks, kale, garlic, rhubarb, figs, tofu, sesame seeds, chia seeds, almonds, flaxseeds, carob powder, plant milks and tofu products fortified with calcium
Chromium	• Keeps blood sugar levels balanced. • Normalizes hunger, reduces cravings.	Broccoli, green beans, tomatoes, romaine lettuce, apples, grapes, whole wheat, barley, oats, brewer's yeast
Iron	• Helps take oxygen to all tissues and muscles. • Supports cells' energy metabolism.	Spinach, olives, chard, sesame seeds, pumpkin seeds, sunflower seeds, cashew nuts, chickpeas, kidney beans, peanuts, soybeans, lentils, rice bran, wheat bran, amaranth, corn, rye, oat bran, parsley, chives, spirulina, agar agar seaweed

Magnesium	• Keeps bones and teeth strong. • Needed for energy production. • Helps muscles to relax. • Supports the nervous system. • Reduces inflammation.	Spinach, chard, bananas, figs, prunes, apricots, watermelon (with seeds), soybeans, black beans, quinoa, rice, wild rice, wheat, buckwheat, amaranth, oat bran, teff, agar agar seaweed, spirulina, yeast extract, pumpkin seeds, flaxseeds, Brazil nuts, sunflower seeds, sesame seeds, almonds, cashew nuts
Manganese	• Important to keep bones, cartilage, tissues, and nerves healthy. • Has a role in normal brain function. • Helps balance blood sugar. • Essential for insulin production.	Celery, lemongrass, leeks, raspberries, okra, lima beans, grapes, beetroot, garlic, peppers, pineapple, blueberries, rice, wheat, teff, rye, oats, agar agar seaweed, hazelnuts, pine nuts, pecans, macadamia nuts, chestnuts, pumpkin seeds, peanuts, soy beans
Potassium	• Keeps muscles and nerves working properly. • Supports heart and kidney function. • Keeps blood pressure balanced.	Sweet potato, potatoes, tomato, beetroot, banana, butternut squash, parsley, sweet peppers, chives, apricots, bananas, peaches, lychee, prunes, raisins, medjool dates, figs, pears, avocado, plantain, grapefruit, apples, palm hearts, onions, shiitake mushrooms, rice, wheat, rye, buckwheat, oat bran, quinoa, amaranth, barley, black beans, soybeans, yeast extract, spirulina, agar agar seaweed, chestnuts, pumpkin seeds, sunflower seeds, flaxseeds, almonds, hazelnuts, brazil nuts, cashew nuts, pine nuts, pistachios
Selenium	• Needed for the production of glutathione, the body's own powerful antioxidant. • Supports normal thyroid function.	Found in most plant foods but especially brazil nuts, sesame seeds, wheat, shiitake mushrooms, soybeans.

Zinc	• Helps the immune system fight infections. • Keeps skin healthy - fights acne. • Needed for sense of taste and smell. • Important for male reproductive health.	Sesame seeds, pumpkin seeds, lentils, chickpeas, cashew nuts, quinoa, oats, wheat bran, wild rice, shiitake mushrooms, agar agar seaweed, watermelon seeds, soy beans, peanuts
Phytonutrients and antioxidants	• Neutralize free radicals. • Slow down the aging process. • Protect DNA. • Reduce the risk of disease.	Brightly colored fruits and vegetables Herbs: rosemary, coriander, oregano, parsley, mint, thyme Spices: ginger, garlic, turmeric, cinnamon, cumin

APPENDIX 2:

GUT-FRIENDLY FOODS AND WAYS TO ADD THEM TO YOUR DIET

KOMBUCHA (FERMENTED TEA):
This is probably the easiest probiotic to add to your diet. Just drink a glass or two every day. When you buy kombucha, check the label to make sure it is raw, unpasteurized, and does not contain any artificial additives or added sweeteners.

SAUERKRAUT (FERMENTED CABBAGE):
You can make this at home or find it in health food shops. Make sure it is raw and unpasteurized, otherwise it won't contain beneficial bacteria. Sauerkraut is wonderful on top of a salad, added to a hummus wrap, or piled on top of a rice cake or oat cracker with smashed avocado.

KIMCHI (FERMENTED CABBAGE WITH GINGER, GARLIC, CHILI):
Like sauerkraut but with an Asian twist and plenty of heat. Complements stir-fried dishes, can be enjoyed added to salads, or added to your wraps and sandwiches.

COCONUT KEFIR
(DAIRY-FREE FERMENTED MILK ALTERNATIVE MADE WITH KEFIR GRAINS):
You'll find coconut kefir in health food shops. Add it to smoothies, pour it on granola or fruit, or drink it on its own.

MISO (FERMENTED RICE PASTE):
Try white miso in dressings and marinades. It has a mild savory flavor that lifts ingredients out of bland and plonks them decidedly into tasty. You can also use miso paste to make Asian noodle dishes. Dark miso has a more pronounced savory flavor - a little goes a long way!

TEMPEH OR NATO (FERMENTED SOY BEANS):
Tempeh is delicious marinated in soy sauce, ginger, and garlic, and fried in a little coconut oil. You can also cut it into chunks and add it to stews and curries for extra protein. It has a subtle, slightly nutty taste. Nato has a very strong flavor and isn't for the faint-hearted.

PICKLES (LACTO-FERMENTED VEGETABLES):
Crunchy, sharp and tangy, picked vegetables are great as a side to any meal, or added to wraps and salads.

MEAL IDEAS TO GET YOU STARTED

PLANT-BASED BREAKFASTS

Chia pudding made with almond milk and topped with berries	High in fiber, protein and healthy fats (chia seeds) High in antioxidants (berries) BONUS: can be made in batches for quick & easy breakfast.
Home-made buckwheat granola with coconut yogurt and fruit	High in fiber and protein (buckwheat) Good source of healthy fat (coconut) Good source of antioxidants (fruit) BONUS: can be made in batches for quick & easy breakfast.
Scrambled tofu, fried mushrooms, roasted tomatoes, home-made baked beans	High in protein and fiber (tofu, beans) Good source of vitamins and antioxidants (mushrooms, tomatoes)
Two slices of seeded sourdough bread with peanut butter and banana	Good source of complex carbs (seed bread, banana) Complete protein from combining seeds & legumes (seeds & peanut butter) Source of healthy fats (peanut butter)
Overnight oats topped with stewed apples and almond butter	Complex carbs and fiber (oats) Good source of antioxidants and fiber (apples) Healthy fats, fiber and protein (almond butter) BONUS: you can make enough for 2 or 3 breakfasts in advance.
Superfood smoothie with spinach, banana, apple, oats, hemp seeds, plant milk	High in fiber (oats, spinach, hemp seed) Complex carbs (oats, banana) Healthy fats and protein (hemp seeds) BONUS: you can go wild with your smoothies - try kale, berries, oats, tropical fruit, coconut milk, cacao, peanut/almond butter... the possibilities are endless.

PLANT-BASED LUNCHES/DINNERS

Buddha bowl: black rice, avocado, chickpeas, steamed broccoli, grated beetroot, tahini dressing	Healthy fats (avocado, tahini) Antioxidants (beetroot, broccoli) Protein (chickpeas) Fiber (all ingredients)
Buddha bowl: quinoa, grated carrot, diced celery, massaged kale, beetroot hummus, toasted seeds	Healthy fats (seeds) Antioxidants (carrot, kale, celery) Protein (hummus, quinoa, seeds) Fiber (all ingredients) BONUS: there's nothing easier than a Buddha bowl meal. Just freestyle with whatever veg you have in your fridge!
Stir fried vegetables (mange tout, mushrooms, tenderstem broccoli, leeks) with buckwheat noodles and a peanut tamari sauce	Antioxidants (broccoli, leeks...) Complex carbs (noodles) Complete protein (combination of buckwheat and peanuts) Healthy fats (peanuts) Fiber (all ingredients)
Parsnip tabbouleh (parsnip rice with finely diced cucumber, celery, mint, lemon juice, sunflower seeds)	Antioxidants (cucumber, celery, mint) Healthy fats (sunflower seeds) Complex carbs (parsnips) Fiber (all ingredients)
Tamari and ginger marinated tempeh with spinach and coconut black rice	Protein and fermented food (tempeh) Complex carbs (black rice) Antioxidants (ginger, spinach) Healthy fats (coconut) Fiber (all ingredients)
Lentil & coconut dhal with buckwheat	Protein (lentils, buckwheat) Complex carbs (buckwheat) Antioxidants (spices, ginger, garlic, onion) Fiber (all ingredients)
Bean & vegetable stew with polenta or whole grain pasta	Protein (beans) Antioxidants (onions, garlic, vegetables) Complex carbs (polenta or whole grain pasta) Healthy fats (olive oil) Fiber (all ingredients)
Roasted root veg (beetroot, sweet potato, parsnips....) and quinoa salad with lemon dressing	Complex carbs (root veg) Antioxidants (sweet potato, beetroot) Protein (quinoa) Healthy fat (olive oil dressing) Fiber (root veg, quinoa)

PLANT-BASED SNACKS

Oat, raisin & pumpkin seed cookie	Complex carbs (oats, raisins) Healthy fats and protein (seeds) Fiber (all ingredients)
Coconut, oat & ginger cookie	Complex carbs (oats) Healthy fats (coconut) Antioxidants (ginger) Fiber (all ingredients)
Energy ball - coconut & mango; oat, peanut & cacao nibs; almond & date...	Complex carbs (oats, dates) Healthy fats and protein (nuts, seeds) Antioxidants (cacao nibs) Fiber (oats, dates, seeds) BONUS: add a tablespoon of vegan protein powder or superfood powders like maca for added goodness.
Oat crackers with nut butter	Complex carbs (oats) Healthy fats (peanut butter) Complete protein (combining grains and legumes) Fiber (oats, peanut butter)
Home-made turmeric buckwheat granola with plant milk	Healthy fats (coconut oil, seeds) Complex carbs (oats) Protein (buckwheat) Antioxidants (turmeric) Fiber (oats, buckwheat)
Dark chocolate	Antioxidants and healthy fats (cacao)

ACKNOWLEDGMENTS

This second book in my *REBEL VEGAN LIFE* series was another labor of love. And bringing a book to life takes a small village, and I am grateful to my team of rebels for helping with its birth.

Firstly, I am indebted to my editor, Gareth Clegg, whose creativity and patience kept me focused. He fine-tuned every aspect of this book and even found time to design the layout. Thank you for believing in this book and me from the beginning.

My copywriter, Elaine Hutchison, made me look good and rallied my spirits when I most needed it. Thank you.

It was a thrill and honor to have one of my heroes, Victoria Moran, write a special foreword for *REBEL VEGAN LIFE*. She was a massive influence in my life and this book. I am eternally grateful for her generous support and endorsement of my work.

Writing this book involved many specialists in helping research and interpreting some of my medical and scientific research. Special thanks to my nutritionist Mel for patiently explaining all the health implications and becoming a friend in the process. I am also grateful for the generous guidance, advice, and encouragement from Dr. Laura Freeman from Plant-Based Health Online.

I am incredibly thankful to my talented design team: Marco, for designing my logo, Jelena, for bringing my book cover concept to life, and my dear neighbor, Cathy, for her striking illustrations that give my text extra force and beauty.

Lara Schirkhorschidi helped develop my recipes and elevate them into culinary art. We had a lot of fun taste testing, and now I want our own cooking show.

My life runs smoothly most days, thanks to my assistant Ruth. Thank you so much for your patience and for being my representative on Earth.

Research and writing can be a lonely process. But I was strengthened and sustained throughout it by my family and friends around the world. Even my earliest friends from my childhood in Canada were still there for me. Special thanks to Kathy, who gave fantastic advice on my cover and brand. Charlie Brown always gave the best inspiration and ideas. Jason always kept me positive and hydrated. My beautiful sisters, Karen, Debbie, and Laura, were the first to believe in me.

To Emma, who was my rock and held my hand throughout the process, I can't thank you enough. Without this foundation, every page in this book would be blank.

And finally, thanks to all my fellow rebels, fighting for compassion and truth.

ABOUT THE AUTHOR

TODD SINCLAIR is the author of the *REBEL VEGAN LIFE* series.

A passionate travel expert, activist, podcaster, writer & speaker for the vegan cause, Todd currently lives his best *REBEL VEGAN LIFE* based in London.

If not writing in his favorite city, you can find him exploring the world—perfecting his cooking in Southeast Asia, trekking volcanoes, or scuba diving, all while promoting plant-based living and putting veganism on the map.

Find out more about *REBEL VEGAN* at the website
RebelVeganLife.com

Or on Social Media

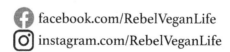

facebook.com/RebelVeganLife
instagram.com/RebelVeganLife

ALSO BY TODD SINCLAIR

REBEL VEGAN LIFE:
A RADICAL TAKE ON VEGANISM FOR A BRAVE NEW WORLD

———————

REBEL VEGAN LIFE:
A PLANT-BASED NUTRITION & BEGINNERS GUIDE

———————

REBEL VEGAN LIFE:
THE ULTIMATE TRAVEL GUIDE FOR
PLANT-BASED ADVENTURES IN A BRAVE NEW WORLD

REFERENCE NOTES

00 - INTRODUCTION
1 https://www.azquotes.com/quotes/topics/truth.html
2 https://www.peta.org.uk/issues/animals-not-eat/meat-health/
1 https://freefromharm.org/animal-farmer-turned-vegan/howard-lyman-former-beef-and-dairy-farmer/ and https://www.youtube.com/watch?v=94QaCbytLEY

01 - COMPASSIONATE REVOLUTION
1 https://www.azquotes.com/quote/907397
2 https://quotlr.com/author/john-eliot
3 www.cowspiracy.com/facts
4 https://www.cowspiracy.com/facts
5 https://www.nationalgeographic.com/animals/article/animals-science-medical-pain
6 https://en.wikipedia.org/wiki/Western_pattern_diet
7 https://mercyforanimals.org/blog/pigs-are-intelligent-and-sensitive-so-why/
8 [Sources: Joy, Melanie (2011) [2009]. Why We Love Dogs, Eat Pigs, and Wear Cows: An Introduction to Carnism. Conari Press, p. 9. ISBN 1573245054. Andhttps://en.wikipedia.org/wiki/Carnism]
9 https://indianexpress.com/article/lifestyle/life-style/go-vegetarian-save-wildlife-planet-sir-david-attenborough-7148660/
10 www.livekindly.co/inconvenient-sequel-overlooks-truth
11 www.washingtonpost.com/climate-environment/2021/08/29/how-climate-change-helped-make-hurricane-ida-one-louisianas-worst/
12 https://apnews.com/article/fires-environment-and-nature-california-wildfires-a7df1b3939dfaa5114fb47d78cfea57f
13 www.siwi.org/facts-and-statistics/6-food-and-agriculture-and-bioenergy
14 https://www.undispatch.com/bad-news-world-will-begin-running-water-2050-good-news-not-2050-yet/
15 www.animalmatters.org
16 https://www.sailorsforthesea.org/programs/ocean-watch/ocean-dead-zones
17 https://seashepherd.org/2015/09/29/if-the-ocean-dies-we-all-die/
18 https://nutritionstudies.org
19 https://www.pcrm.org/good-nutrition/nutrition-information/health-concerns-about-dairy
20 https://www.goodreads.com/quotes/162579-i-choose-not-to-make-a-graveyard-of-my-body
21 https://www.ncbi.nlm.nih.gov/pmc/articles/PMC5035214/
22 http://apps.who.int/iris/bitstream/handle/10665/112642/9789241564748_eng.pdf
23 https://www.pewtrusts.org/en/research-and-analysis/articles/2020/01/16/antibiotic-sales-for-animal-agriculture-increase-again-after-a-two-year-decline
24 https://assets.publishing.service.gov.uk/government/uploads/system/uploads/attachment_data/file/773065/uk-20-year-vision-for-antimicrobial-resistance.pdf
25 https://www.goodreads.com/author/quotes/149151.Francis_of_Assisi
26 https://kidadl.com/articles/best-justice-quotes-to-fight-for-equality
27 https://foodprint.org/issues/what-happens-to-animal-waste/ and US Environmental Protection Agency. "Basic Information about Nonpoint Source (NPS) Pollution. EPA, (n.d.). Retrieved May 31, 2018 from https://www.epa.gov/nps/basic-information-about-nonpoint-source-nps-pollution
28 https://theecologist.org/2020/may/05/vegan-diet-can-stop-future-pandemics
29 www.cdc.gov/onehealth/basics/zoonotic-diseases.html
30 https://www.cowspiracy.com/facts

02 - VEGANOMETRY
1 https://www.heromovement.net/blog/vegan-quotes/
2 https://www.heromovement.net/blog/vegan-quotes/
3 https://www.health.harvard.edu/staying-healthy/cutting-red-meat-for-a-longer-life
4 The Standard American Diet (SAD), also known as the standard Western diet, is a pattern of eating is generally characterized by high intakes of meat, dairy products, eggs, fried foods, refined grains, and refined sugars, with low intakes of vegetables, fruits, whole grains, legumes, nuts and seeds.
5 https://pubmed.ncbi.nlm.nih.gov/29634829/ andhttps://www.hvst.com/posts/the-leading-cause-of-both-death-and-disability-in-the-u-s-is-the-american-diet-oNRTZkgk
6 http://www.dresselstyn.com/site/
7 https://www.google.com/search?q=tobacco+advert+for+pregnant+women&tbm=isch
8 https://www.thelancet.com/journals/lancet/article/PIIS0140-6736(12)62089-3/fulltext
9 https://www.who.int/news-room/q-a-detail/cancer-carcinogenicity-of-the-consumption-of-red-meat-and-processed-meat

10   https://www.dietaryguidelines.gov/sites/default/files/2020-12/Dietary_Guidelines_for_
      Americans_2020-2025.pdf
      https://health.gov/our-work/food-nutrition/previous-dietary-guidelines/2015;https://health.
      gov/our-work/food-nutrition/previous-dietary-guidelines/2010 andhttps://health.gov/our-
      work/food-nutrition/previous-dietary-guidelines/2005
11   https://www.heromovement.net/blog/vegan-quotes/
12   https://www.ncbi.nlm.nih.gov/pmc/articles/PMC2121650/
13   https://www.jwatch.org/na52921/2020/12/23/red-meat-and-cardiovascular-risk-revisited
14   https://www.ahajournals.org/doi/10.1161/01.ATV.0000038493.65177.94
15   https://jamanetwork.com/journals/jama/fullarticle/200732
16   Sex Robots & Vegan Meat: Adventures at the Frontier of Birth, Food, Sex and Death - by Jenny
      Kleeman
17   https://epi.grants.cancer.gov/diet/foodsources/top-food-sources-report-02212020.pdf
18   https://academic.oup.com/ije/article-abstract/49/5/1526/5743492
19   https://www.eurekalert.org/pub_releases/2019-10/aoa-mcr101819.php
20   https://pubmed.ncbi.nlm.nih.gov/22882905/
21   https://www.fda.gov/media/136671/download
22   https://www.who.int/health-topics/cardiovascular-diseases#tab=tab_1
23   https://pubmed.ncbi.nlm.nih.gov/29496410/
24   https://www.who.int/health-topics/cancer#tab=tab_1
25   https://acsjournals.onlinelibrary.wiley.com/doi/full/10.3322/caac.21440
26   https://www.ncbi.nlm.nih.gov/pmc/articles/PMC3048091/
27   https://www.who.int/news-room/facts-in-pictures/detail/6-facts-on-obesity
28   https://www.who.int/health-topics/obesity#tab=tab_1
29   https://pubmed.ncbi.nlm.nih.gov/32922235/
30   https://www.who.int/health-topics/diabetes#tab=tab_1
31   https://pubmed.ncbi.nlm.nih.gov/29948369/
32   https://www.who.int/news-room/fact-sheets/detail/dementia
33   https://pubmed.ncbi.nlm.nih.gov/34214643/
34   https://www.ncbi.nlm.nih.gov/pmc/articles/PMC6846186/
35   https://www.worldometers.info/coronavirus/coronavirus-death-toll/
36   https://nutrition.bmj.com/content/4/1/257
37   https://www.goodreads.com/author/quotes/35040.Neal_D_Barnard
38   https://www.heromovement.net/blog/vegan-quotes/
39   https://www.thediabetescouncil.com/45-alarming-statistics-on-americans-sugar-
      consumption-and-the-effects-of-sugar-on-americans-health/
40   https://www.dietaryguidelines.gov/sites/default/files/2020-12/Dietary_Guidelines_for_
      Americans_2020-2025.pdf#page=31
41   https://www.nhs.uk/live-well/eat-well/how-does-sugar-in-our-diet-affect-our-health/
42   https://www.ncbi.nlm.nih.gov/pmc/articles/PMC4244242/
43   https://www.ncbi.nlm.nih.gov/pmc/articles/PMC3614697/
44   https://bmjopen.bmj.com/content/6/3/e009892
45   https://www.ncbi.nlm.nih.gov/pmc/articles/PMC5938543/
46   https://pubmed.ncbi.nlm.nih.gov/2836348/
47   https://pubmed.ncbi.nlm.nih.gov/22889895/
48   https://pubmed.ncbi.nlm.nih.gov/28507982/
49   https://pubmed.ncbi.nlm.nih.gov/22538314/
50   https://pubmed.ncbi.nlm.nih.gov/28229641/
51   https://www.euroweeklynews.com/2021/03/15/lebanon-introduces-worlds-first-hospital-
      serving-only-vegan-food/
52   https://www.sciencedirect.com/topics/engineering/acute-inflammation
53   https://www.ncbi.nlm.nih.gov/books/NBK493173/
54   Sources for footnotes:https://www.bda.uk.com/resource/british-dietetic-association-
      confirms-well-planned-vegan-diets-can-support-healthy-living-in-people-of-all-ages.html
      https://pubmed.ncbi.nlm.nih.gov/19562864/
      https://pubmed.ncbi.nlm.nih.gov/12778049/
55   Sources:https://nutritionstudies.org/the-china-study-3-lessons-we-need-to-know/https://
      pubmed.ncbi.nlm.nih.gov/9860369/ andhttps://www.pnas.org/content/115/15/3804

03 - VEGAN NUTRITION

1   https://www.drmcdougall.com/
2   https://www.drfuhrman.com/
3   https://medlineplus.gov/ency/article/002222.htm
4   https://www.ncbi.nlm.nih.gov/books/NBK56068/table/summarytables.t4/?report=objectonly
5   http://www.whfoods.com/genpage.php?tname=foodspice&dbid=79
6   https://www.huffingtonpost.co.uk/entry/beyond-meat-impossible-burger-healthy_l_5d164ad
     1e4b07f6ca57cc3ed
7   https://www.huffingtonpost.co.uk/entry/beyond-meat-impossible-burger-healthy_l_5d164ad
     1e4b07f6ca57cc3ed

8   http://www.whfoods.com/genpage.php?tname=foodspice&dbid=52
9   http://www.whfoods.com/genpage.php?tname=foodspice&dbid=56
10   http://www.whfoods.com/genpage.php?tname=foodspice&dbid=58
11   http://www.whfoods.com/genpage.php?tname=foodspice&dbid=142
12   http://www.whfoods.com/genpage.php?tname=foodspice&dbid=98
13   http://www.whfoods.com/genpage.php?tname=foodspice&dbid=84
14   http://www.whfoods.com/genpage.php?tname=foodspice&dbid=11
15   http://www.whfoods.com/genpage.php?tname=foodspice&dbid=20
16   http://www.whfoods.com/genpage.php?tname=foodspice&dbid=81
17   http://www.whfoods.com/genpage.php?tname=foodspice&dbid=53
18   http://www.whfoods.com/genpage.php?tname=foodspice&dbid=128
19   http://www.whfoods.com/genpage.php?tname=foodspice&dbid=9
20   http://www.whfoods.com/genpage.php?tname=foodspice&dbid=45
21   http://www.whfoods.com/genpage.php?tname=foodspice&dbid=122
22   http://www.whfoods.com/genpage.php?tname=foodspice&dbid=38
23   http://www.whfoods.com/genpage.php?tname=foodspice&dbid=62
24   https://www.huffingtonpost.co.uk/entry/beyond-meat-impossible-burger-healthy_l_5d164ad
     1e4b07f6ca57cc3ed
25   https://www.ncbi.nlm.nih.gov/books/NBK22436/
26   https://www.ncbi.nlm.nih.gov/pubmed/17921363
27   https://pubmed.ncbi.nlm.nih.gov/28462631/
28   https://www.nature.com/articles/1602940
29   https://www.medicalnewstoday.com/articles/319176#what-are-the-benefits-of-fiber
30   https://www.helpguide.org/articles/healthy-eating/high-fiber-foods.htm
31   https://www.pcrm.org/good-nutrition/nutrition-information/fiber
32   https://www.pcrm.org/good-nutrition/nutrition-information/the-carbohydrate-advantage
33   https://www.health.harvard.edu/heart-health/how-its-made-cholesterol-production-in-your-
     body
34   https://pubmed.ncbi.nlm.nih.gov/27784848/
35   https://www.fda.gov/media/135274/download
36   https://pubmed.ncbi.nlm.nih.gov/31442459/
37   https://www.iarc.who.int/featured-news/media-centre-iarc-news-glyphosate/
38   https://en.wikipedia.org/wiki/Canola_oil
39   https://www.ncbi.nlm.nih.gov/pmc/articles/PMC3335257/
40   https://www.pcrm.org/good-nutrition/nutrition-information/lowering-cholesterol-with-a-
     plant-based-diet

41   https://www.nih.gov/news-events/news-releases/nih-human-microbiome-project-defines-
     normal-bacterial-makeup-body
42   https://pubmed.ncbi.nlm.nih.gov/32432868/
43   Mao, Q., Manservisi, F., Panzacchi, S., Mandrioli, D., Menghetti, I., Vornoli, A., Hu, J. (2018). The
     Ramazzini Institute 13-week pilot study on glyphosate and Roundup administered at human-
     equivalent dose to Sprague Dawley rats: effects on the microbiome. Environmental health: a
     global access science source, 17(1), 50. doi:10.1186/s12940-018-0394-x -https://www.ncbi.
     nlm.nih.gov/pmc/articles/PMC5972442/
44   https://ods.od.nih.gov/factsheets/Omega3FattyAcids-Consumer/
45   https://www.cochranelibrary.com/cdsr/doi/10.1002/14651858.CD003177.pub3/full
46   https://pubmed.ncbi.nlm.nih.gov/29355094/
47   https://www.jandonline.org/article/S2212-2672(13)01113-1/fulltext
48   https://rarediseases.org/rare-diseases/anemia-megaloblastic/
49   https://pubmed.ncbi.nlm.nih.gov/18606874/
50   https://www.vegansociety.com/resources/nutrition-and-health/nutrients/vitamin-b12
51   https://www.doctorklaper.com/
52   https://www.ncbi.nlm.nih.gov/pmc/articles/PMC3449318/
53   https://www.hsph.harvard.edu/nutritionsource/calcium/
54   http://www.whfoods.com/genpage.php?tname=nutrient&dbid=45
55   Le CH. The prevalence of anemia and moderate-severe anemia in the US population (NHANES
     2003-2012). PLoS One. 2016 Nov 15;11(11):e0166635.https://journals.plos.org/plosone/
     article?id=10.1371/journal.pone.0166635
56   Nadia M. Bastide, Fabrice H.F. Pierre and Denis E. Corpet. "Heme Iron from Meat and Risk of
     Colorectal Cancer: A Meta-analysis and a Review of the Mechanisms Involved." Cancer Prev
     Res February. (2011): 177-184.
57   https://ods.od.nih.gov/factsheets/Iron-HealthProfessional/
58   http://www.whfoods.com/genpage.php?tname=nutrient&dbid=70
59   https://ods.od.nih.gov/factsheets/Zinc-HealthProfessional/
60   https://www.mja.com.au/journal/2013/199/4/zinc-and-vegetarian-diets
61   https://ods.od.nih.gov/factsheets/Zinc-HealthProfessional/
62   http://www.whfoods.com/genpage.php?tname=nutrient&dbid=115
63   https://pubmed.ncbi.nlm.nih.gov/15971062/

64 https://www.bmj.com/content/356/bmj.i6583
65 https://pubmed.ncbi.nlm.nih.gov/21310306/
66 https://ods.od.nih.gov/factsheets/VitaminD-HealthProfessional/
67 https://ods.od.nih.gov/factsheets/VitaminD-HealthProfessional/
68 https://www.bbc.com/news/health-57968651
69 https://pubmed.ncbi.nlm.nih.gov/9787730/
70 https://pubmed.ncbi.nlm.nih.gov/32788355/
71 https://www.nature.com/articles/s41591-020-01209-1

04 - REBEL VEGINNERS GUIDE

1   https://foodrevolution.org/blog/plant-based-yogurt/?utm_source=sfmc&utm_medium=email&utm_campaign=blo-2021&utm_content=plant-based-yogurt
2   https://www.virtua.org/articles/prevent-and-reverse-heart-disease-with-a-plant-based-diet
3   https://www.healthline.com/health-news/quitting-junk-food-produces-similar-withdrawals-as-drug-addiction#What-junk-food-does-to-your-brain andhttps://www.sciencedirect.com/science/article/abs/pii/S0195666318306196
1   https://www.psychologytoday.com/us/blog/animals-and-us/201412/84-vegetarians-and-vegans-return-meat-why

05 - EATING IN, EATING OUT, AND COMING OUT

1   https://vegnews.com/2021/5/vegan-meal-kits
2   DeGeneres, Ellen - The Funny Thing Is... (2003)
3   https://www.researchgate.net/publication/317768313_Discrimination_Against_Vegans
4   https://journals.sagepub.com/doi/abs/10.1177/1368430215618253
5   https://journals.sagepub.com/doi/abs/10.1177/1368430215618253

06 - BEYOND DIET

1   https://www.peta.org/features/expert-quotes-reasons-animal-testing-unreliable
2   https://www.peta.org/features/expert-quotes-reasons-animal-testing-unreliable
3   https://www.unep.org/news-and-stories/story/putting-brakes-fast-fashion
4   https://www.worldwildlife.org/stories/the-impact-of-a-cotton-t-shirt
5   de Janvry, Alain; McIntosh, Craig; Sadoulet, Elisabeth (July 2015). "Fair Trade and Free Entry: Can a Disequilibrium Market Serve as a Development Tool?". The Review of Economics and Statistics. 97 (3): 567–573. doi:10.1162/REST_a_00512. S2CID 27543341. Andhttps://en.wikipedia.org/wiki/Fair_trade_debate
6   https://bcorporation.net/
7   https://grist.org/article/nasas-james-hansen-on-hacked-emails/
8   https://www.nestle.com/aboutus/overview/ourbrands
9   https://www.coca-colacompany.com/brands

07 - STAYING MOTIVATED AND INSPIRED

1   https://www.brainyquote.com/topics/secret-quotes
2   https://www.brainyquote.com/topics/secret-quotes
3   https://www.brainyquote.com/topics/secret-quotes
4   https://winstonchurchill.org/resources/quotes/page/3/
5   https://www.goodreads.com/work/quotes/100074-d-o-d-j-ng
6   https://kidadl.com/articles/open-minded-quotes-to-open-yourself-up-to-the-world
7   https://kidadl.com/articles/open-minded-quotes-to-open-yourself-up-to-the-world
8   https://kidadl.com/articles/open-minded-quotes-to-open-yourself-up-to-the-world
9   https://en.wikipedia.org/wiki/John_Quincy_Adams
10 https://libquotes.com/neal-d-barnard/quote/lbx9r7i
11 https://www.goodreads.com/author/quotes/149151.Francis_of_Assisi
12 https://www.greatsayings.net/sayings-about-not-giving-into-temptation/
13 https://healingwithplants.us/2018/02/former-president-bill-clinton-healed-heart-disease-with-a-plant-based-diet
14 https://getlighthouse.com/blog/john-wooden-quotes-leadership-manager/
15 https://www.growthengineering.co.uk/55-quotes-about-learning/
16 https://www.growthengineering.co.uk/55-quotes-about-learning/
17 https://www.futurekind.com/blogs/vegan/10-vegan-celebrities
18 https://www.garyfox.co/inspirational-quotes/
19 https://www.azquotes.com/quote/811759
20 https://www.futurekind.com/blogs/vegan/10-vegan-celebrities
21 https://www.garyfox.co/inspirational-quotes/
22 https://www.goalcast.com/socrates-quotes
23 https://elated.co.za/vegan-quotes/
24 https://www.garyfox.co/inspirational-quotes/
25 https://www.azquotes.com/author/19347-Colleen_Patrick_Goudreau

26 @lizzo/tiktok

08 - FINAL THOUGHTS

1   https://www.euronews.com/2020/04/01/the-best-way-prevent-future-pandemics-like-coronavirus-stop-eating-meat-and-go-vegan-view
2   https://www.ncbi.nlm.nih.gov/pmc/articles/PMC7721435/
3   https://pubmed.ncbi.nlm.nih.gov/31728489/
4   https://www.worldwatch.org/node/6294 andhttps://mercyforanimals.org/blog/this-new-study-is-further-proof-that-going/
5   https://ireland-calling.com/george-bernard-shaw-quotes-vegetarianism/
6   https://www.goodreads.com/quotes/13287-you-see-things-you-say-why-but-i-dream-things

11 - APPENDICES

1   Information sourced fromhttps://nutritiondata.self.com/
2   Info sourced fromhttp://www.whfoods.com andhttps://nutritiondata.self.comhttps://www.goodreads.com/quotes/13287-you-see-things-you-say-why-but-i-dream-things

Made in United States
North Haven, CT
10 December 2021